D0362963

HAIRDRESSING FOR NVQ LEVEL 3

PAT DUDLEY AND BOB WOODHOUSE

Hodder & Stoughton

A MEMBER OF THE HODDER HEADLINE GROUP

Orders: please contact Bookpoint Ltd, 130 Milton Park, Abingdon, Oxon OX14 4SB. Telephone: (44) 01235 827720. Fax: (44) 01235 400454. Lines are open from 9.00–6.00, Monday to Saturday, with a 24 hour message answering service. You can also order through our website www.hodderheadline.co.uk.

British Library Cataloguing in Publication Data
A catalogue record for this title is available from the British Library

ISBN 0 340 802952

First Published 2003
Impression number   10 9 8 7 6 5 4 3 2 1
Year   2007 2006 2005 2004 2003

Copyright © 2003 Pat Dudley and Bob Woodhouse

All rights reserved. No part of this publication may be reproduced or transmitted in any form or by any means, electronic or mechanical, including photocopy, recording, or any information storage and retrieval system, without permission in writing from the publisher or under licence from the Copyright Licensing Agency Limited. Further details of such licences (for reprographic reproduction) may be obtained from the Copyright Licensing Agency Limited, of 90 Tottenham Court Road, London W1T 4LP.

Cover images occur courtesy of: Serge Krouglikoff/Stone and Getty Images; Nick Koudis, Photodisc/Getty Images; and Digital Vision/Getty Images.
Typeset by Fakenham Photosetting Limited, Fakenham, Norfolk
Printed in Italy for Hodder & Stoughton Educational, a division of Hodder Headline Plc, 338 Euston Road, London NW1 3BH

CONTENTS

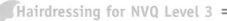

Acknowledgements

The authors would like to thank the following: Kingston College students and staff, Ray Dudley, Indola, IBC and Capital Hair and Beauty

For the reproduction of photographs the publishers would like to thank the following:

West Kent College, Tonbridge, Kent for providing facilities for David Guy, Technical Director, and Bob Woodhouse.

Figures 3.2, 3.4, 3.7, 3.20, 3.21, 10.9, 10.10 courtesy of The Science Photo Library

Use of HABIA hairdressing standards by kind permission of:

HABIA, Fraser House, Nether Hall Road, Doncaster, South Yorkshire, DN1 2PH (Telephone: 01302 380000, fax 01302 380028 Email: enquiries@ habia.org.uk Website: www.habia.org.uk

If acknowledgement has been inadvertently omitted, the omission will be rectified at the earliest possible opportunity.

ABOUT THIS BOOK

This book covers topics relating to selected units for the NVQ 3 Hairdressing New Standards. There are two main routes in NVQ/SVQ qualifications at Level 3 in Hairdressing. These are:

- Hairdressing Level 3
- Barbering Level 3.

The above qualifications are intended to provide a progression route from Level 2 Hairdressing. Both of these Level 3 awards have a mandatory and optional unit structure that cater for general hairdressing and barbering with special 'routes' for African Caribbean hairdressing and specialist technical work.

Many new units have been introduced, which should be of interest to new entrants to the profession and will also provide a Continuous Professional Development (CPD) route for many existing hairdressers who are keen to extend their skills and qualifications. Nine units must be completed for the full NVQ/SVQ (i.e. four mandatory and five optional).

This book is intended to cover the two main structures. Individual units can be awarded, which will be certificated on successful completion of a Record of Achievement.

For lecturers, each unit can be delivered as a short course. There are a lot of generic requirements that can be used to encourage students to take more than one unit eventually leading to a full award if required. The book also covers information required for the following awards:

- City and Guilds/Edexcel NVQ 3 Hairdressing
- City and Guilds/Edexcel NVQ 3 Barbering
- City and Guilds NVQ 3 Diploma in Hairdressing (6915)
- City and Guilds NVQ 3 Diploma in Barbering (6913)
- Advanced Modern Apprenticeship in Hairdressing.

INTRODUCTION

How to use this book

You may use this book either as a reference text, a self-study aid or a support for guided learning. As a reference book the contents list and detailed index will support you in locating specific references or information. The book may be used as part of an integrated programme of professional development. The text will provide you with guidance in competent performance and good practice. Illustrations provide support to your understanding and to illustrate practical tasks. At the beginning of each chapter the relevant elements of the level 3 Hairdressing and Barbering awards are stated.

Within each chapter there is guidance in activities that will provide evidence of your competence and/or knowledge for the award.

How to undertake assessment of skills

National Vocational Qualifications are achieved through the confirmation of your competence, knowledge and understanding across a range of specified criteria and situations. They require evidence of current competence that is generated mainly through real work activity. The most frequently used method of assessment for hairdressing skills is by the observation of these activities and their results as they occur in the salon. This is effective in confirming that the competence is current, that of the candidate and relevant to the part of the award being assessed.

Alternatively, evidence of your performance can be provided through the presentation to your assessor of evidence of your activities by:

- testimony from your work colleagues
- your personal statement
- your responses to questioning
- case study
- previous qualifications, relevant experience and achievement.

There are guidelines in good and acceptable practice in assessment and the awarding body often prescribes what methods are particularly suitable for particular parts of the award.

As a National Vocational Qualification candidate you will negotiate the assessment of your competence with your allocated assessor. Your assessor will have current relevant hairdressing skills and have a recognised assessor qualification. You will normally be guided towards undertaking assessment when it is expected that you are competent.

Before undertaking assessment you will plan with your assessor how and when this will take place. The detail agreed will include:

- how evidence will be presented – most frequently by you undertaking a task that is observed by your assessor
- the task that will produce appropriate evidence
- the units and elements of the award against which you are to be assessed
- when the assessment will occur – this may be a single event or a number of events that occur over a period of time
- when progress or achievement will be reviewed.

It is important that you fully understand what you are expected to do before you undertake assessment. During an observation of your performance you will be encouraged, by your assessor, to undertake the task while they are unobtrusive

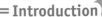

but able to observe effectively. As soon as is practicable following the assessment your assessor will provide you with feedback, and confirm and record the outcome of the assessment.

If you feel that the assessment has been undertaken inappropriately or the assessment decision is unfair you should discuss this with your assessor. Assessment centres have guidelines in how to make an appeal if you believe you have been unfairly treated.

How to achieve the award

You will achieve the full National Vocational Qualification award when your assessor has confirmed your competence in all of the mandatory units of the award and the required optional units and when this has been quality assured through the process of internal verification. This includes sampling the assessment process including the support that you have received, the appropriateness of the decisions made and the prompt processing of the records.

You may wish to gain recognition for specific units of the award, in preference to the full National Vocational Qualification. A certificate of unit credit may be claimed for units that are completed.

Further and complementary qualifications

There is a range of National Vocational Qualifications that are relevant to the hairdressing industry and can support your further development and recognise the achievement of competence. You may wish to consider their appropriateness for your continued development.

Some NVQs apply to roles often undertaken in close relationship to hairdressing, for example Beauty Therapy. Appropriate awards that confirm competence and are not specific to hairdressing but are applicable to a wide range of organisations include Customer Service, Management and Business Development. Achievement of National Vocational Qualifications is dependant upon you, the candidate, being able to present evidence of competent work-based performance and therefore requires you to be in the job role or at least in a position to undertake that role.

If you aspire to a role but are not yet within that role or do not have access to the role you may consider alternative qualifications that are based upon a level of achievement through examination of knowledge and simulated or non-work-based activity. These are known as Technical Certificates. The achievement of these qualifications can provide an indication of the potential for performance when placed into the job role.

Role of HTB and HABIA in developing and maintaining the standards

The authors recognise the contribution that the Hairdressing Training Board (HTB) has made in the identification and development associated with the national standards. The HTB is part of the National Training Organisation – The Hairdressing and Beauty Industry Authority (HABIA). This is the independent employer-led sector organisation recognised by the Department for Education and Skills for working with the hairdressing and beauty therapy sectors and government across education and training throughout the whole of Great Britain. It is mainly concerned with:

- identifying shortages in skills and the training needs for beauty and hairdressing
- influencing the provision of education and careers guidance
- developing the occupational standards, including NVQs/SVQs
- advising on training arrangements and its provision
- effectively communicating with employers and key partners to implement their plans.

As national standards of competence and the qualifications they are based upon are reviewed to ensure that they continue to be relevant to the needs of the industry, the structure and content of National Vocational Qualifications and Scottish Vocational Qualifications may differ from the descriptions within this text. You are advised to seek clarification and confirmation from your assessor.

THE AWARD UNIT STRUCTURE

Mandatory Units	Unit Title	Main Outcomes	Compulsory/ Optional
G1	Ensure your own actions reduce risks to health and safety	1 Identify hazards and evaluate the risks in your workplace 2 Reduce the risks to health and safety in your workplace	Compulsory
G6	Promote additional products or services to clients	1 Identify additional products or services that are available 2 Inform clients about additional products or services 3 Gain client commitment to using additional products or services	Compulsory
G9	Provide hairdressing consultation services	1 Identify clients' needs and wishes 2 Analyse the hair, skin and scalp 3 Make recommendations to clients 4 Agree services with your client	Compulsory
G10	Support customer service improvements	1 Use feedback to identify potential customer service improvements 2 Contribute to the implementation of changes in customer service 3 Assist with the evaluation of changes in customer service	Option Group 2 Hairdressing Barbering
G11	Contribute to the financial effectiveness of the business	1 Contribute to the effectiveness of the business using and monitoring resources 2 Meet productivity and development targets	Option Group 2 Hairdressing Barbering
H19	Provide shaving services	1 Maintain effective and safe methods of working when shaving 2 Prepare the hair and skin for shaving 3 Shave hair	Option Group 1 Barbering
H20	Design a range of facial hair shapes	1 Maintain effective and safe methods of working when cutting facial hair 2 Create a range of facial hair shapes	Option Group 1 Barbering
H21	Create a variety of looks using barbering techniques	1 Maintain effective and safe methods of working when cutting hair 2 Create a variety of looks for men	Compulsory Barbering
H22	Design and create patterns in hair	1 Maintain effective and safe methods of working when creating designs in hair 2 Plan and agree hair pattern designs with your client 3 Create patterns in hair	Option Group 1 Barbering
H24	Develop and enhance your creative skills	1 Plan and design a range of images 2 Produce a range of creative images 3 Evaluate your results against the design plan objectives	Option Group 1 Hairdressing Barbering

Mandatory Units	Unit Title	Main Outcomes	Compulsory/ Optional
H25	Style and dress hair to create a variety of looks	1 Maintain effective and safe methods of working when styling hair 2 Style and dress hair creatively	Option Group 1 Hairdressing
H26	Style and dress long hair	1 Maintain effective and safe methods of working when styling long hair 2 Creatively dress long hair	Option Group 1 Hairdressing
H27	Create a variety of hairstyles using a combination of cutting techniques	1 Maintain effective and safe methods of working when cutting hair 2 Cut hair to create a variety of looks for women	Compulsory for Hairdressing not for Barbering
H28	Provide colour correction services	1 Maintain effective and safe methods of working when correcting hair colour 2 Determine the problem 3 Plan and agree a course of action to correct colour 4 Correct colour	Option Group 1 Hairdressing
H29	Perm hair to create a variety of looks	1 Maintain effective and safe methods of working when perming hair 2 Prepare for perming 3 Create a variety of permed effects	Option Group 1 Hairdressing
H30	Colour hair using a variety of techniques	1 Maintain effective and safe methods of working when colouring hair 2 Prepare for colouring 3 Create a variety of colouring effects 4 Resolve basic colouring problems	Option Group 1 Hairdressing
H32	Contribute to the planning and implementation of promotional activities	1 Contribute to the planning and preparation of promotional activities 2 Implement promotional activities 3 Participate in the evaluation of promotional activities	Option Group 2 Hairdressing Barbering
H34	Provide face massaging services	1 Maintian effective and safe methods of working when providing face massage services 2 Prepare the skin for massage services 3 Carry out face massage services	Option Group 1

UNIT G1 ENSURE YOUR OWN ACTIONS REDUCE THE RISKS TO HEALTH AND SAFETY IN THE SALON

1 Identify hazards and evaluate the risks in your workplace

2 Reduce the risks to health and safety in your workplace

CHAPTER CONTENTS

- Risk
- Risk Assessment
- Health and Safety Risk Assessment
- COSHH Assessment
- Personal Appearance and Hygiene
- Good Practice in Hygiene and Safety in the Salon
- Legislation

- Emergency Procedures
- Good Practice in Salon Security
- Responsibilities for Personal Possessions and the Salon
- Further Development Activities
- Review Questions
- Additional Information
- Activity

Introduction

Everyone at work has a legal obligation not to intentionally or knowingly put themselves or others at risk either by their actions or omissions. This places considerable responsibility on you, the hairdresser, as you work not only with colleagues but also with clients/members of the public. There are a number of legislative regulations that specify these responsibilities; some are the responsibility of the salon owner (or person responsible for the management of the salon) and some are the responsibility of all employees.

As a member of the salon team, and with a level of supervisory or management responsibility, you will have responsibility for ensuring that appropriate procedures are in place, and that people are aware of these and comply with them. Ignorance of these responsibilities is not a mitigating factor. You should set an example of good practice to others who work with you.

Risk

This section will provide you with guidance in good practice as a member of staff and a person with supervisory responsibility within the hairdressing salon. This includes supervisor's roles and responsibilities for good working practices, safety within the hairdressing salon and strategies that may be used to support you in fulfilling these. There is an overview of some legislation that is applicable to safety within the hairdressing salon and indicates how they may apply.

Supervisory responsibilities in ensuring safe working practices – responsibilities to staff and clients

Those with management and supervisory roles have responsibilities for supporting safe working practices. These practices will help to make the salon commercially successful, while at the same time providing a safe environment for staff and clients. In order to fulfil the requirements of this role you need to ensure that all staff are fully aware of the expectations that you have of them and their performance. When staff first join your team provide them with guidance in safe working practices – do not assume that this knowledge already exists. Remember, salons may have varying practices and expectations.

Consistently act as a role model for the practices that you expect. Staff will look to you for examples of good practice and to provide guidance in standards of behaviour. This includes examples of good practice at times of stress or high pressure of work. Within the salon assume a level of corporate responsibility; should a situation occur that falls outside your area of responsibility do not ignore this but either deal with it or report it to the appropriate person. If you are in doubt, promptly report the situation to your manager.

If unsure of the expectations that your manager has of you, discuss this with them. You may have specifically stated activities that you are required to undertake, for example ensuring that adequate supplies of protective gloves are maintained within the salon. Your activities may be broader and stated as accountabilities, for example ensuring that safe working practices are observed within the salon.

Identify risk

There is a certain amount of risk-related activity within the salon environment. First of all you need to develop an awareness of potential hazards in order to reduce risk. First ask yourself how you would carry out the following and maintain safe practices.

Write down how you achieve the following:

- Maintain effective and safe methods when cutting hair.
- Maintain effective and safe methods of working when perming and neutralising hair.
- Maintain effective and safe methods of working when colouring hair.
- Maintain safe working practices within the salon.
- Monitor and maintain salon security.
- Maintain effective and safe methods of working when thermally styling and relaxing hair.
- Maintain effective and safe methods of working when styling hair.

Once you have written down some answers you will need to research the following:

- Your supervisory responsibilities in ensuring safe working practices – responsibilities to staff and clients.
- The salon's health and safety policies and procedures.
- The salon's expectations of staff personal appearance and hygiene.
- Local bye-laws from your local council related to hairdressing.
- Good practice in hygiene and safety in the salon.
- What makes good practice.

Risk assessment

This is an assessment of any potential hazards within the hairdressing salon. Employers are required to undertake an assessment of risk within the salon regularly (recommended at least every six months or whenever working practices change).

Health and safety risk assessment

First review your salon and its practices for potential hazards. These may include low door openings, shelves that project, trailing electrical leads, and use of open razors (this list is not exhaustive). It can often be beneficial for more than one person to work on this task.

● Identified risks should be prioritised, considering who is at risk, the nature of the risk, and the likelihood of the risk.

● Alternative practices should be considered to reduce or remove the risk, options considered and implemented if realistic.

● An action plan should be developed to implement remedial action.

In all cases the preferred action is to remove the risk. When this is not practicable then actions to reduce the risk, either through changes and improvements, training and warnings should be provided. Having identified a risk it is important that a level of corrective or preventative action is taken.

Repetitive strain injuries

These injuries can occur as the result of prolonged work activity. To reduce the risk ensure that you adopt correct working practices and vary your workload.

As a person with supervisory responsibility you should encourage people to work correctly, for example holding tools correctly, using the correct techniques, and varying work. Staff may require training and coaching.

COSHH assessment

The Control of Substances Hazardous to Health (COSHH) regulations require an assessment to be made of every substance that is used within the salon. A substance is considered to be hazardous if it may cause harm if inhaled, ingested, comes in contact with the skin, is absorbed through the skin, is injected into the body or enters the body via skin abrasions.

All substances used should be assessed for potential hazards. Within the hairdressing salon products including perm lotion, hydrogen peroxide and oxidation tint can be hazardous.

Guidance in the potential for hazard of a product will usually be given in data sheets available from manufacturers. It is an employer's responsibility to determine if there are risks in the use or misuse of the substance in their salon. If a risk is identified you should determine who is at risk and the nature of the risk. Preventative or corrective action should be undertaken to remove or reduce the risk. If the risk cannot be reduced and protection from the potential consequences cannot be provided, you should make a decision as to whether the risk is acceptable. Training may be required for staff in the correct use of substances. Staff should be informed of any risks and any remedial action to be undertaken in the case of accident.

COSHH assessment should be undertaken when any new products are introduced to the salon. Staff new to the salon will require training in the safe use of products and corrective actions. A chart, indicating potential hazards, corrective and remedial action that can be seen and understood by all staff, can help to communicate the message.

Remember: Some products may appear to be without risk, but when assessed have a risk if user guidelines are not followed.

Remember: A substance on its own may be quite harmless but when mixed with others may become hazardous. This should be considered within a risk assessment.

First Aid

It is advisable that staff should go through some type of first aid training and update on a regular basis. As you are working in a customer-led industry you never know when you might have to deal with an accident or emergency.

In the salon find out the following information if you haven't been told in induction:

● What to do in case of an emergency

● Who is the first aider at work?

● Where the first aid box is located

● How to report accidents and to whom

Be aware of occupational hazards such as:

● Chemical spillages causing burns to the scalp and skin

● Burns to the scalp and skin from hot water

● Chemicals and products splashing into the eyes

● Electric shocks

● Allergic reactions

● Choking

● Cuts from sharp instruments and how to dispose of them appropriately

Then there are a whole variety of incidents that you might be able to address e.g.

● Fainting

● Heart attack

● Deep cuts and abrasions due to a fall etc.

● A hypo from a person suffering from diabetes

Again these are just a few examples. It is better to be safe and report these in the first instance to a first aider who has been trained and is up to date with the latest techniques. What would be far more useful is to undergo some form of training yourself.

You should only carry out first aid treatments if you are qualified to do so. Even with basic incidents (such as minor cuts) you should know how to respond correctly to avoid risks such as HIV or Hepatitis.

Personal appearance and hygiene

Appearance

Your appearance will project an image to clients. First impressions can set the tone of your professional relationship with clients. Many salons have a predetermined style of acceptable or required dress for work. This usually ensures that a corporate image is projected (see Unit H31 – Promotions).

Clean, easily maintained protective clothing should be worn when working within the hairdressing salon. Local authority bye-laws may require protective clothing to be worn. Within this industry the precise nature of this clothing is interpreted widely. Clothing should, for example, protect you from damage or injury from hair cuttings or spillage of products you or others use, and protect your client by not

> *Remember: As a supervisor it is more efficient to provide clear guidance in good practice before the occurrence. Prevention is often more easily applied than a cure.*

encouraging cross contamination. Regular laundering of clothing will not only maintain a level of personal hygiene but also remove spilt chemicals, some of which can be simultaneously combustible (self igniting).

Shoes should provide support and protection. Your toes and the sides of your feet need to be protected from spillages and dropped items, particularly those that may be sharp or heavy. You will be standing for lengthy periods during the working day, so to prevent unnecessary fatigue and posture abnormalities your shoes should provide support, i.e. having heels that are not too high. Supervisors often have responsibility to provide guidance in appropriate clothing for staff to wear within the salon. If specialist protective clothing is provided when appropriate, ensure that staff correctly use this. Failure to support staff in these practices can lead to periods of staff absence due to illness or injury.

Hygiene

You will be working in close proximity with your clients and colleagues and it is important that your personal hygiene is maintained. Body odour and strong smells within the confined space of a hairdressing salon can be very oppressive for clients and colleagues. Key points for personal hygiene:

- Bathe frequently and use appropriate anti-perspirant and/or deodorants.

- If you perspire heavily, reapply deodorants and consider washing during the day.

- Wear clean, aired clothing.

- Avoid using overly heavy or strong fragrances.

- Register for regular dental care.

Remember: Odours on the breath from strongly spiced food or smoking can be unpleasant for others.

While working with clients, exposed open cuts or sores should be covered with a waterproof dressing.

As a supervisor or manager you will have responsibilities in guiding others in appropriate hygienic practices. If neglected, this may have an adverse affect on the salon's activity either by producing an unpleasant atmosphere or by causing staff illness. Set an example to others through your own good practice. Consider briefing new staff, within their induction, about your expectations and relevant salon rules. While it can be embarrassing to all concerned to provide feedback about adverse personal hygiene, when necessary all staff have a corporate responsibility to the salon to do this. It can be less kind to a colleague not to tell them and allow them to continue to work in ignorance.

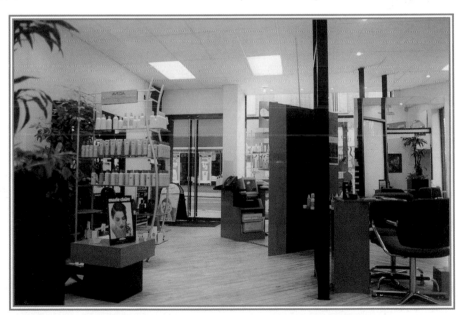

Figure 1.1 A safe and hygienic salon environment

Good practice in hygiene and safety in the salon

The hairdressing salon can provide the perfect environment for bacteria growth and cross infection. The maintenance of high standards of hygiene are essential. Your clients will

Remember: Your local authority may have bye-laws that identify codes of hygienic practices.

have awareness, heightened by the current increased focus on safety and hygiene, and will expect to see evidence of your hygiene procedures.

The salon should be frequently and regularly cleaned. This task can be made easier and often more effective if surfaces and furniture are washable. At times there has to be a trade-off between the look of a salon and its ease of cleaning. When selecting furniture remember to consider how it may be cleaned.

All hairdressing salons need effective equipment and practices to ensure that tools used on clients are clean and sterile and that the risk of cross infection is kept to as low a level as possible.

Instruments and equipment

Whenever equipment is used on more than one client there is a risk of cross infection. To reduce this risk all items should be cleaned and, when relevant, sterilised between use. This includes small portable equipment as well as larger fixed equipment.

Immediately following use all equipment must be cleaned and sterilised. Equipment should always be left ready for use. Equipment left unclean may contaminate other equipment, as well as being a risk to you and your colleagues who may accidentally come in contact with them.

Equipment cleaning

Always consult manufacturer's guidance before cleaning equipment. Some equipment may be cleaned by using warm soapy water, by total immersion or by wiping with a dampened cloth. Electrical equipment should **not** normally be immersed or soaked in water. A moistened cloth may be more appropriate. Equipment that is best not made wet may be cleaned using specialised cleaning agents, often spirit based.

Remember: Consult with manufacturer's guidelines – damage may be caused through incorrect use of cleaning materials.

When cleaned all items should be allowed to dry and, if small, placed in a covered container to reduce the risk of contamination.

Sterilisation

Sterilisation can be achieved using chemicals, rays or heat. For sterilisation to be effective items must be clean and dry before the process begins. Grease left on the surface of tools can reduce the effectiveness of the process and contaminate the sterilising product.

Chemical disinfectants

These are effective only if used in the correct strength. Once the disinfectant has become soiled it is no longer effective. There are a range of chemical sterilising products available including liquids, moist wipes and aerosol sprays. Some liquid products require dilution using clean water; others are used at their full strength. Always follow manufacturer's

Remember: Some plastics are adversely affected by the application of certain chemicals.

guidelines in use and the suitability for use. Many sterilising liquids require the items to be immersed in the solution and to remain immersed for a period of time. Maintain the strength of the solution as, through use and time, its effectiveness can diminish. Manufacturers provide guidelines relating to this. Avoid dust and particles that can contaminate the product, as they will reduce its effectiveness. Manufacturers often provide specialised containers in which to hold the chemical and the tools immersed in it.

Some sterilising chemicals are applied using a clean pad. These are particularly suitable for use on tools that should not be immersed in liquid. Remember that only those areas that the chemical contacts will be sterilised.

> *Remember: Take care when disposing of empty aerosol containers; do not store containers near heat.*

Vapours

Vapours are usually formaldehyde based. They are used in cabinets and again quite popular in salons as they are easy to use. Tools must be cleaned thoroughly before placing them in to the cabinet, turned on all sides and exposed to the vapours so that they work effectively.

Radiation

Ultraviolet light cabinets may be used for sterilising. The cabinets usually have reflective interior surfaces and a specialist electrical bulb that produces ultraviolet light rays. Those surfaces that are exposed to the light rays are sterilised. So that all areas are treated, ensure that items in the steriliser are rotated. Avoid overfilling the steriliser cabinet, as those items in shadow will not be sterilised. Turn

> *Remember: Unprotected exposure to ultraviolet light can be injurious. Always follow manufacturer's guidelines in safe working practice.*

tools part way through the process to ensure effective exposure to the ultraviolet light. Manufacturers provide guidelines on minimum period of exposure to ensure effective sterilisation. The effectiveness of ultraviolet bulbs deteriorates with use; consult specialist service agents for advice and guidance.

Heat

Dry heat

This can be done by placing items in very high temperatures in the oven (usually towels, sheets, etc). Some barbers use pre-packed towels that have been prepared and wrapped in this way. While dry heat can be used to sterilise equipment that has a tolerance to heat, within the hairdressing salon moist heat is most frequently used.

Moist heat

Moist heat can be applied by boiling items in water for 20 minutes, or by immersing them in steam and under pressure in an autoclave. The autoclave operates in the same way as a pressure cooker. Moist heat at high pressure is produced within an autoclave. A small volume of water is placed in the autoclave and the equipment to be sterilised is placed within a container that rests slightly above. The autoclave is sealed shut and the heat source turned on. The autoclave heats to a pre-determined temperature and remains at this for a set period of time. High pressure enables the water to boil and produce steam at a higher temperature than that which is otherwise achieved in the hairdressing salon, usually 121°C. This technique is suitable only for equipment that is not adversely affected by heat and steam.

> *Remember: Do not open an autoclave during its operation or before it has cooled for its recommended period as this can result in dangerous escape of high pressure, high temperature steam. Allow the autoclave and its contents to cool, remove the lid, remove the contents and store them ready for use. Always follow the manufacturer's guidelines in correct use. The outside surface of an autoclave can become very hot while in use. Avoid contact with it during this period.*

Legislation

The following Acts have been passed by Parliament to protect workers and clients in industry, including the hairdressing industry.

- The Health and Safety at Work Act 1974

- Control of Substances Hazardous to Health Regulations (COSHH)1988
- Personal Protective Equipment (PPE) at Work Regulations 1992
- Workplace (Health, Safety and Welfare) Regulations 1992
- Health and Safety (Display Screen Equipment) Regulations 1992
- Manual Handling Operations Regulations 1992
- Provision and Use of Work Equipment Regulations (PUWER) 1992
- Electricity at Work Regulations 1989
- Reporting Injuries, Diseases, and Dangerous Occurrences Regulations (RIDDOR) 1985

The Health and Safety at Work Act 1974

All people in the workplace have a legal responsibility not to intentionally put themselves or others at risk by their actions or omissions. Employers have a duty of care to employees and others in the salon or those affected by the work of the salon. Employees should comply with an employer's reasonable requests in pursuance of this Act.

Within your hairdressing salon this will include:

Employers' responsibilities:

- providing instruction in safe working of equipment, for example scalp steamers, hair clippers, etc
- providing instruction in safe working practices with chemicals, for example handling of perm lotion, bleach, hydrogen peroxide, etc
- ensuring that equipment is safe for use, for example having effective procedures for checking the safety of electrical tools and for reporting breakages.

Employees' responsibilities:

- using protective equipment provided, for example using protective gloves when handling oxidation tint and perm lotion
- responding to guidance in safe working practices, for example not storing hydrogen peroxide on high shelving with the risk of spillage on to the user, and promptly clearing up any spillage on the floor or work surfaces
- participating in training for safe working provided by the employer.

This is not an exhaustive list.

Control of Substances Hazardous to Health Regulations 1988 (COSHH)

This Regulation requires employers to consider potential hazards to people exposed to substances in the salon. This includes undertaking assessments of substances for potential hazards. For those that are identified as potentially hazardous, alternatives for use that are less hazardous should be considered and safe working procedures identified and communicated to all those likely to be affected.

Within your hairdressing salon this will include:

- whenever practicable using lower volume strengths of hydrogen peroxide
- ensuring employees wear protective gloves when applying oxidation tint
- providing instruction in procedures to apply in case of injury or accident involving hazardous products
- storing products safely and securely. Products that may react if mixed with each other should not be stored together
- if bulk products are decanted into smaller containers, this should be done using suitable containers that are clearly labelled.

This is not an exhaustive list.

Personal Protective Equipment (PPE) at Work Regulations 1992

This Act requires employers to provide suitable protective equipment, free of charge, to employees. Employees must report to their employer any loss or damage of these provisions.

Within your hairdressing salon this will include:

- protective gloves for use when handling oxidation tint, perm lotion, bleach, etc
- protective clothing, aprons, etc. for use when applying hair colour.

This is not an exhaustive list.

Workplace (Health, Safety and Welfare) Regulations 1992

The Regulation applies to all workplaces and sets minimum standards of facilities and the provision of safe premises in which to work.

Within your hairdressing salon this will include: the salon including room dimensions and work area, floors, passageways, stairs, lighting, effective salon ventilation, and reasonable working temperatures and its monitoring. Salon facilities including toilets, washing, drinking water and accommodation for clothes.

This is not an exhaustive list.

Health and Safety (Display Screen Equipment) Regulations 1992

The Regulations describe minimum standards for workstations that have display screens (computers, etc) and their use. It states minimum requirements for breaks away from the screen for users, appropriate eye and eyesight tests for regular users, and the provision of training in correct use.

This is not an exhaustive list.

Manual Handling Operations Regulations 1992

This Regulation requires that employers assess an individual's capability to carry or move stock/equipment, and to provide guidance in safe working practices.

Within your hairdressing salon this will include:

- providing suitable trolleys for moving large or heavy equipment or boxes
- instructing employees how to safely handle large or heavy items.

This is not an exhaustive list.

Provision and Use of Work Equipment Regulations (PUWER) 1992

This regulation requires an employer to provide equipment that is suitable for its use and properly maintained. All staff using this equipment should be trained in its safe use.

Electricity at Work Regulations 1989

This Regulation requires employers to maintain all electrical equipment and installations in a safe condition. Employees have a responsibility to report any faulty electrical equipment.

Reporting Injuries, Diseases, and Dangerous Occurrences Regulations (RIDDOR) 1985

This Regulation requires the occurrence of listed industrial-related diseases and disorders to be reported to the Health and

Safety Inspectorate. The list includes potentially infectious conditions. Accidents occurring at work that require hospitalisation or long periods of absence from work must also be reported. Currently absences from work for more than three days caused by an accident or injury must be reported.

Emergency procedures

Evacuation in emergency procedures

Your salon will have fire and evacuation procedures. The local authority will license your salon and may issue procedures. All staff should be aware of procedures before the need to use them arises. Events that may lead to evacuation of the salon include:

- fire
- gas escape (remember not to use naked flame, turn electrical switches, or use electrical machinery including mobile telephones in an area of gas escape – these may ignite the gas)
- flood
- suspicious people and packages
- dangerous incident.

Procedures will require prompt action and will state:

- who, within the salon, to inform of a fire or emergency
- how to recognise a fire or smoke alarm signal
- how the emergency services are contacted
- how the salon is to be evacuated, the exit routes, and where and to whom workers should report when the evacuation is completed. This will include the location of the pre-determined assembly points where those who exit the salon in an emergency should congregate. These points will be close to the salon but not in a position that will place people at risk or create an obstruction to the emergency services
- how clients and visitors are to be supported during these events.

As a person with supervisory responsibility for staff you will have a duty to ensure they are fully aware of these emergency procedures and that they are complied with.

Fire fighting equipment and its correct use

Ensure that you are aware of the location, within the salon, of all fire fighting equipment, such as fire extinguishers and fire blankets.

If a fire is minor it may be possible to take corrective actions. These actions may include the use of the correct fire extinguisher. Fire extinguishers or their labels are colour coded to differentiate between their contents and intended use. Take care to ensure that the correct choice is made. Most appliances are accompanied with guidance in their correct and appropriate use. Do not attempt any corrective action if it puts yourself or others at risk.

If possible, turn off any electrical or gas appliances, and close windows before vacating the salon.

Appropriate fire extinguishers

Water extinguishers

These are suitable for use on fires involving materials such as wood, paper and fabrics. Water is a fast and efficient means of extinguishing these materials. It works by having a rapid cooling effect, so that insufficient heat remains to sustain burning and so continuous ignition ceases.

Foam spray extinguishers

Foam spray extinguishers (AFFF – Aqueous Film Forming Foam) are ideal for multi-risk situations involving wood, paper, textiles and flammable liquids such as oils, spirits, greases, fats and certain plastics. The blanketing effect of foam spray gives rapid flame knock down, which smothers the flame and thus prevents re-ignition of flammable vapours by sealing the surface of the solution.

Powder extinguishers

Powder extinguishers are suitable for use on fires involving wood, paper, fabrics, flammable liquids, flammable gases (propane and butane) and electrical hazards. The multi-purpose powder interferes with the combustion process and provides rapid fire knock down.

Carbon dioxide extinguishers – CO_2

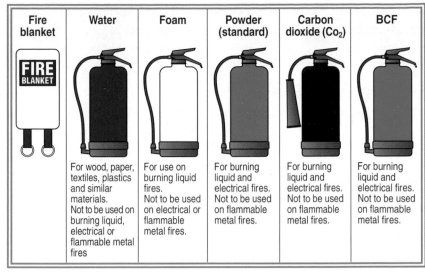

Figure 1.2 Appropriate fire extinguishers

Carbon dioxide extinguishers are suitable for fires involving flammable liquids and electrical hazards. The non-corrosive and non-conductive qualities of CO_2 make it an ideal choice for dealing with fires involving electrical equipment and machinery.

Class of Fire	Water	Foam	Powder	CO_2
Paper, wood, textiles and fabric	■	■	■	
Flammable liquids		■	■	■
Flammable gases			■	■
Electrical equipment			■	■
Transport/domestic, e.g. boats, cars, caravans, the home		■	■	

Good practice in salon security

Every member of the hairdressing salon should accept a level of personal responsibility in the maintenance of the salon's security. The level of responsibility will vary according to your salon's requirements. However, it is reasonable to expect every employee to take reasonable care of the salon's security.

Those aspects of security at the most basic level include reporting apparent breaches of security to the person responsible. Do not place the salon security at risk by, for example:

- failing to check the credentials of all people entering the premises
- leaving cash on display at unattended reception areas
- leaving cash drawers open and unattended
- placing small items of stock or equipment in areas from which they may readily be illegally removed
- leaving emergency exit doors open

- blocking or locking emergency access and exit points
- interfering with any equipment provided for salon security.

If you are in doubt about your responsibilities, discuss this with your supervisor or manager.

As a supervisor or manager you will wish to provide guidance in good practice to your team. Setting a good example by your own actions is a good starting point but you will need to formalise systems and procedures for:

- cashing up
- recording stock holdings, usage and requirements
- storing client and staff personal belongings
- locking and unlocking the salon premises.

Responsibilities for personal possessions and the salon

Stated procedures provide guidance to staff concerning the salon's methods and these procedures can be developmental tools for staff. Systems ensure that the appropriate people use procedures. When reviewing your salon's procedures consider the following:

Cash

Avoid keeping high levels of cash on the premises and in particular within the till. At regular intervals remove large denomination currency notes and large volumes of cash from the till. Ensure that monies held within the till reconcile with that expected from the client numbers and planned treatments. You will require procedures for providing refunds and the use of cash from the till to make petty cash payments. Some salons restrict access to money within the till to specified persons only. This is recommended.

Equipment

Your salon requires procedures and systems for maintenance of equipment. This includes regular checks for standards of cleanliness, damage or breakage, and regular electrical safety (Portable Appliance Testing PAT) checks undertaken by a qualified electrician. Ensure staff who use their own electrical equipment in the salon have this equipment electrically tested. Many organisations do not allow personal electrical equipment to be used on their premises, as they are unable to effectively monitor their safety.

Information

If your salon holds personal details of either clients or staff on computer, password protected access should be considered to maintain the security of this confidential information. (See also page 44 Data Protection Act 1998.) Personal Information held in other systems, i.e. manual, must also be kept securely. The salon will need to consider who will be provided with access to this information, in particular any person outside of the salon. Information about the performance of the salon, client appointments, client numbers, cash takings, and staff performance should be stored securely.

People

If you have people within your salon in vulnerable situations you need adequate security at entry to the salon. You may have areas of the salon to which only staff have access.

Possessions

You will, very likely, be accommodating personal possessions of clients and staff. You need secure places for the storage of clients' clothing and possessions while undergoing treatment. Your salon may have a stated policy relating to the level of responsibility accepted for clients' possessions. Staff need space to store clothes while working. Secure space is also required for staff to store personal items that have to be removed while at work.

Premises

Your salon, its fabric, fixtures and fittings require security. You will need to make these secure when not in use. This will include adequate facilities to lock the premises and deter illegal entry. Specialist or high-value items may require additional security. Failure to take reasonable care of the security of the premises may invalidate any insurance protection.

Stock

Rotation of stock will help to reduce its deterioration. It is most usual to rotate stock so that items that were received first are used first. This process is sometimes known and First In First Out (FIFO) and helps to reduce the risks of stock wastage due to deterioration. Stock must be stored securely and safely. Flammable stock must be stored appropriately. Regular and random checks on stock levels can support effective monitoring of stock use and any loss. Effective stock control includes reconciling actual stock use with the level of recorded business activity, forecasting future stock needs, rotating stock to avoid deterioration, and avoiding unnecessary stock purchases. Avoid putting displays of stock in areas that may encourage opportunistic theft; for example, near to public entrances or areas where people may remain unsupervised.

Tools

To reduce risks of cross infection all equipment should be kept in a clean, hygienic condition. The salon should ensure that there is adequate equipment available to allow for the maintenance of hygiene.

Further development activities

This will also help you towards the Technical Certificate.

Exam revision

Remember, legalisation and regulations change and you must ensure you have all current information. This can be achieved by linking to information services including relevant hairdressing employer organisations, local government agencies and local commerce organisations.

Review Questions

1 *State three key points for personal hygiene relating to minimising risk.*

2 *State three ways that tools may be sterilised and how that will minimise risk.*

3 *Who has responsibility for health and safety and risk assessment within the hairdressing salon?*

4 *What is COSHH and why is it so important to adhere to in the salon?*

5 *What is the minimum period of absence from work, resulting from an accident at work, that must be reported to the Health and Safety Inspectorate?*

6 *What is the purpose of risk assessment?*

7 *To avoid a gas explosion, what precautions should be taken if a gas leak is discovered?*

8 *State two types of fire extinguishers suitable for use on electrical hazards and equipment.*

9 *State three precautions that can be taken to avoid placing the salon security at risk.*

10 *State four aspects of effective stock control.*

Design a risk assessment form for use in the workplace or centre taking into consideration that it needs to be quick and easy to use.

Additional information
Useful websites

Website Addresses	Content
www.habia.org.uk	Hairdressing and Beauty Industry Authority. Downloads available, including references to other websites
www.bbc-safety.co.uk	Free advice on diseases in hairdressing
www.haircouncil.org.uk	UK statutory body for hairdressing
www.hmso.gov.uk	Legislation and regulations
www.laurandp.co.uk	Educational publications for development of professional hairdressing
www.hse.gov.uk	Health and safety executive
www.trichologists.org.uk	Institute of Trichologists

The evidence from the activities below will cover the Underpinning Knowledge for the Technical Certificate for Advanced Modern Apprenticeships. You will need to take the external test and carry out the practical activities (see: City and Guilds Diploma Hairdressing 6915/6913).

ACTIVITY

Outcome 1
Produce evidence for your portfolio on the following:

- Describe procedures for dealing with an emergency.
- Describe the correct use of fire fighting equipment on different types of fire.
- Describe how and when to carry out basic first-aid treatments.
- Outline the health and safety legislation for Reporting of Injuries, Diseases and Dangerous Occurrences Regulations (RIDDOR) (1985) and explain how they affect the salon.

Outcome 2
- State the employer's responsibility for providing health and safety in the workplace.
- Describe the procedure for carrying out risk assessment of potential hazards in the workplace.
- State why risk assessments are necessary.
- State why it is important to identify potential breaches in security and respond promptly to them.
- Describe the procedures for dealing with different types of security incidents.
- State the importance of hygiene in the salon.

- *Outline the health and safety legislation for the following and explain how they affect the salon:*
  - *The Health and Safety at Work Act (1974)*
  - *The Management of Health and Safety at Work Regulations (1992)*
  - *The Personal Protective Equipment at Work Regulations*
  - *The Provision and Use of Work Equipment at Work Regulations (1992)*
  - *The Control of Substances Hazardous to Health (COSHH) Regulations (1992)*
  - *The Electricity at Work Regulations (1989)*
  - *The Workplace (Health, Safety and Welfare) Regulations (1992)*

Following the above activities, if you are undertaking the Technical Certificate you will need to be assessed on the practical activity pages 40, 41 City and Guilds Level 3 Diploma in Hairdressing.

2 UNIT G6 PROMOTE ADDITIONAL PRODUCTS OR SERVICES TO CLIENTS

1 Identify additional products or services that are available

2 Inform clients about additional products or services

3 Gain client commitment to using additional products or services

CHAPTER CONTENTS

- *Promoting Aftercare Products and Extending Salon Services*
- *Consumer Legislation*
- *Four Steps in Selling*
- *Additional Information*
- *Activity*

Introduction

This unit will give you an awareness of what is required to become successful when promoting products or services to clients. Clients should be given a complete service when attending the salon to ensure they can handle their hair, getting the best out of it. How many times do we hear clients say, 'Well it looks great when the hairdresser does it but I can't get it to look like that'. Ask yourself why that is!

It is important that you give a complete service by discussing a hair maintenance programme for your clients to ensure their hair stays looking good. The following information will help you to understand how to promote products and services, the principles of selling and how to support the

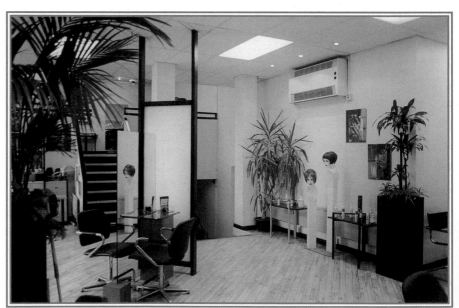

Figure 2.1 Display aftercare products in the salon

selling process by using promotional activities. This information will then help you to develop the skills needed for identifying products and services, informing your client and gaining their commitment.

Promotional activities are most frequently used to develop and improve your salon's business. At times this objective will be quite apparent as the promotional activity will directly increase either the number of clients visiting the salon or the spend that each client makes. Other forms of promotion may have a primary focus of something other than increasing salon business but often, due to the raising of the salon profile or through association with another event, the salon benefits from increased business. These events often include charity fund-raising events, participation in local community activities and helping other local businesses with their charity events. If the promotion is directly connected to improving the salon's business, you will wish to ensure that the activities are carefully planned to meet the promotion objectives and that these plans are implemented effectively to gain the maximum impact.

This chapter will introduce you to a range of potential promotional activities that may be undertaken by your salon independently or in collaboration with others (additional information is included in Chapter 18). It will provide you with a framework for planning and managing these events so that they achieve their objectives in an efficient manner. You will consider the benefits of on-going low-key informal promotions within the salon, regular formal promotional activities and one-off events.

A variety of approaches to promotional activity will be introduced, including ways of supporting the costs of these activities, maximising the impact through publicity, passive and proactive involvement.

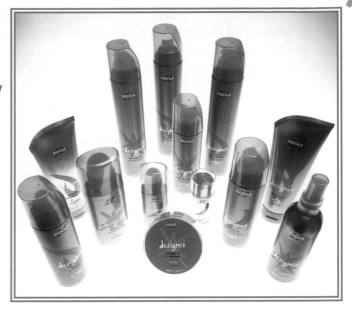

Figure 2.2 A range of aftercare products

Promoting aftercare products and extending salon services

Part of the complete service that the hairdresser provides is that of aftercare procedures and salon services. This potential area of salon business can provide a considerable income that may otherwise be lost to the high street chemist or retail store, or may lead to your client's dissatisfaction with their hair care. Your client will often base their opinion of your hairdressing on how easily they can effectively maintain their hairstyle following the salon visit. They will very rarely object to being offered good advice about how to care for their hair, what products they should use and additional services that create improvement. It is important for you and your team to provide effective advice.

> *Remember: As a trained and qualified hairdresser you are best suited to provide your clients with good advice on aftercare products and services and to promote those that your salon provides.*

For this to occur training will often be required. All staff need to be fully aware of the range of services the salon provides and how they complement each other. They should be aware to whom they should refer clients for more in-depth information and should be encouraged to share with each other information about clients who have expressed interest in particular products or services or have expressed concerns about caring for their hair. Discreet team communication is essential.

Within a whole salon staff team meeting information about the ranges of products and services, their features and benefits, may be shared. Encouraging individuals or small groups to present products or services to the rest of the staff can be developmental for those presenting as well as for those receiving the information. This practice can:

- encourage people to research the products and services they provide
- develop communication skills
- develop presentation skills
- develop a team-sharing culture.

Manufacturer and wholesaler representatives will often provide, without direct cost, briefings to staff about their products' features, benefits and correct use. It is in their interests to ensure the products that they promote are used correctly as this will support customer satisfaction and subsequent sales.

Your clients will value advice and guidance on how to manage their hair following a restyle so that it will look at its best between visits. Your client may not have the skills that you have so do not unrealistically build their expectations. Demonstrate how they may manage their hair using basic home hair care techniques. If you use specific styling products you should have complimentary home hair care products to which your client is introduced. Provide guidance in appropriate products and their use. Some salons embed the cost of home care products within the cost of restyling hair. This ensures that the correct products are available for the client in their home and establishes their use. Salons may provide sample products for clients to enable them to manage their hair in the short term and to introduce a product to them. When your client has belief in a product they will usually continue with its use.

Aftercare support should also be extended to relevant equipment. When a fashion effect that you are promoting requires specialist equipment to support it between salon visits, these should be promoted by the salon. Guide your clients in their correct use. Encourage your client to practise in the salon. You can be assured you have communicated effectively and your client is very likely to be able to manage their hair.

Extend the salon services that you offer to your clients. When a client requires a fashion look that will be enhanced by chemical treatments, such as hair colour, introduce these to them. Do not assume that clients cannot afford these services. Clients often place a high value on the way they look and will value good advice and consider the provision of such advice as an enhancement to the service that the salon provides.

Remember: While your clients will gladly accept good advice and guidance, they will resent being pressured into purchasing goods that they believe are inappropriate.

When discussing a new look with your client consider enhancements at an early stage of the salon visit so that they can be added to the process at the appropriate time. Should your client not wish to take up any of the options presented, they will have time to reflect on them during their visit and may choose to make a future appointment.

Maintain records of the products that your clients purchase or are provided with so that you can follow these up, asking about the success of their use at relevant intervals. This can help to stimulate continuing purchases.

Remember: If your salon retains information about individuals you may be required to register with the Data Protection Commissioner, indicating how this information will be used.

Consumer legislation

You should be aware of the Consumer and Retail Legislation, especially the following:

- The Consumer Protection Act (1987)
- The Consumer Safety Act (1978)
- The Prices Act (1974)
- Trades Description Act (1968 & 1972)
- The Resale Process Act (1964 & 1976)
- The Sale and Supply of Goods Act (1994)
- Cosmetic Product (Safety) Regulations 1989

These Acts protect you and the consumer and it is well worth spending a little time reading through them before you embark on retailing products. If a client isn't happy with their purchase they may want to return the goods. What is your salon policy if this situation arises?

Consumer Protection Act

All products should be safe to use and most manufacturers carry out a lot of research to prevent anything going wrong. However, some clients can be allergic to products thus causing a nasty reaction. It is the responsibility of hairdressers to ensure they are recommending the correct products. This means they should carry out a consultation and try to avoid giving the client a product that isn't suited. Skin tests, strand tests, etc. should be carried out, especially when you are selling the client a colour service. Remember that each type of service may need a different consultation.

Consumer Safety Act

This Act aims to reduce possible risk to consumers from any product that may be potentially dangerous.

Hairdressers deal with chemicals and the public, therefore must ensure they practise safely. In failing to do so they could be sued. I must stress the importance of Consumer Safety and your responsibility as a hairdresser to take all necessary precautions. Read the manufacturer's instructions and ensure you follow some type of consultation that will help you. Read the G9 unit, 'Provide Hairdressing Consultation Services' and the consultation information provided.

What type of consultation do you carry out? Is it thorough enough? If you get the consultation right then the client will more than likely book another service or buy another product. Hairdressers don't sell products just to make money. They sell products to give the client a complete service, and by doing so help the client get the best from their hairdressing services.

Prices Act

The price of products has to be displayed in order to prevent giving a false impression to the buyer.

Pricing structures usually reflect the quality of service or product. They can also reflect how expert the salon team are within the salon environment. The Prices Act 1974 states that if a product or service has been marked up then that is how much the consumer should pay. You may find that some clients will disagree with the price being charged. What are your salon policies on payment discrepancies?

Try to avoid this situation by agreeing the cost before you start. Use the price lists and discuss exactly what is included in the price. Some clients become upset when they think they have been charged too much, and when they weren't aware of the hidden costs, e.g. highlights excluding blow dry. Clients do not always read the small print.

Trades Description Act

Products should not be falsely or misleadingly described orally, in displays or descriptions or in relation to their price, quality and fitness for purpose by advertisements. Since 1972 it is also a requirement to label a product clearly, so the buyer can see where the product was made.

The Trades Description Act requires that consumers should not be misled. You cannot say a product will do something that it won't. As a hairdresser you need to ensure the client is happy and satisfied with their service and products and not mislead them in any way. If a client is not happy, they can complain. Does your salon have a customer complaints procedure and, if so, what is it? If the client is still not happy he/she can take it further by reporting it to the Office of Fair Trading which will investigate the complaint further and possibly take action.

Resale Process Act (1964–1976)

Manufacturers can supply a recommended retail price, but the seller is not obliged to sell it at that price.

Sale and Supply of Goods Act

You, as the seller, must ensure the goods you sell are:

- of satisfactory quality defined as the standard that would be regarded by a reasonable person as satisfactory having taken into account the description of the goods, the price and any other relevant circumstances, and reasonably fit – you must ensure, as a seller, that goods are able to meet what you claim they do.

The Sale and Supply of Goods Act protects the consumer in relation to products that may be out of date or might need to be withdrawn due to the manufacturer's specification as the product is no longer to be sold. When selling products staff may need specific training on how to recommend the products to ensure correct information is given to the consumer. The products should also be stored and displayed appropriately, e.g. out of direct sunlight as it could cause damage.

The information above shows only a few examples and you are therefore recommended to read these Acts in detail and follow if applicable.

Cosmetic Products (Safety) Regulations 2003

These regulations specify chemicals that may not be used in retail cosmetic products and provide safe working practice guidelines for professional use. For example: Perming and straightening products containing 11% Thioglycolic Acid (ready for use) is for professional use only. All perming products containing Thioglycolic Acid must have stated safety instructions.

Four steps in selling

Selling a product or service is a four-step, sequential process:

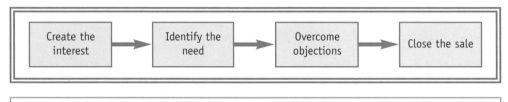

Figure 2.3 The four-step selling process

Create the interest

In most cases your client would not be in the salon if they were completely satisfied with their hair and the way they look. Therefore your client has already indicated their interest in purchasing a service or treatment. Watch out for buying signs that clients may make. These may include:

- questioning about products and services
- looking at and handling retail products and reading their labels
- looking closely at hair or style books.

These signs indicate interest and it is your role to pick up on these and satisfy your client's need. Often your client will be waiting for you to develop their initial demonstration of interest into a consultation with you.

Identify the need

Use your professional expertise to make suggestions about suitable products or services. You may need to use probing questions about your client's hair, preference for hair products and lifestyle to be able to make recommendations about those most suitable for their needs. Use open–ended questions, for example 'how often do you wash your hair', 'which colour do you prefer' or 'is this for use at home or to carry with you'? You can effectively advise your client only when you are aware of their needs through responses to questions and your observations.

You may be asked about your preferences. Be honest but remember that it is only your opinion and may differ from that of others. Allow your client to form their own final judgement based upon the information you have provided, your opinion and their own view. Do not be embarrassed or

Remember: The Trade Descriptions Act 1968 & 1972 prohibits making false claims about what products can do.

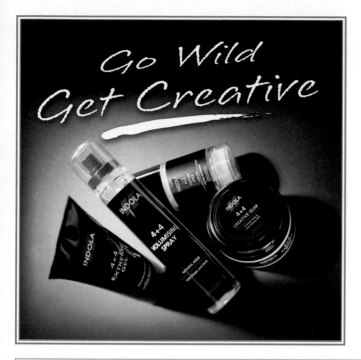

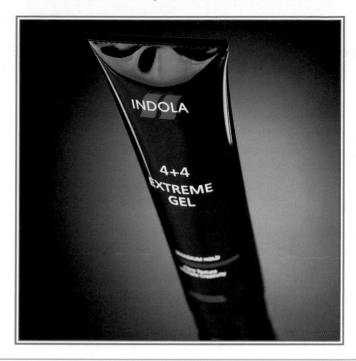

Figure 2.4 Brand image gives products character

apologise for the cost of a product. If the price is appropriate for the product, it should not be a barrier to the sale. Do not assume that a product is too expensive for your client; they may place a high value on themselves and the care of their hair.

Overcome objections

Should your client demonstrate resistance to the sale, find out what the problem is by questioning. Do not take rejection as a personal insult or attribute blame. Do not argue with your client but accept their point of view and outweigh it by calmly outlining the benefit of the product. Break the problem down into its smallest parts and deal with each one in turn. You may need to provide further justification about what the product can do and how it will meet your client's needs. Be prepared to provide more information about the product's features and benefits and to identify alternatives should these be more appropriate. Never be afraid of an objection as this can provide you with the opportunity to promote and confirm the features and benefits of the product. The availability of tester products can support you at this stage providing samples with which to demonstrate and confirm your claims. At this stage the need for a product has already been established; it is now a case of confirming the appropriate product.

Ultimately, the decision to buy rests with your client. The wider the range of aftercare products that you have within the salon and the fuller your knowledge of the products, their features and benefits, the more likely you are to be able to satisfy your client's purchasing needs.

> *Remember: Actively listen to what your client is really telling you within any consultation process.*

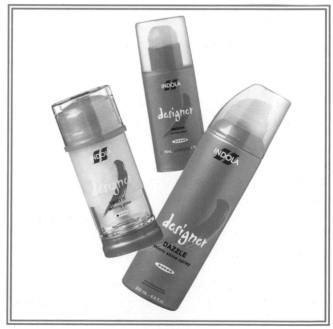

Figure 2.5 Aftercare products come in different ranges

Close the sale

When your client confirms their wish to purchase, close the sale. Your client may confirm acceptance by simply telling you they wish to purchase or you may detect this by their attitude or how they retain the product in their hands. Bring the consultation to a conclusion by either:

- confirming the total client spend
- agreeing which of the products the client is purchasing
- arranging how products will be kept at the salon reception for the client's collection.

Additional information

Useful websites

Website Addresses	Content
www.habia.org.uk	Hairdressing and Beauty Industry Authority. Downloads available including references to other websites
www.bbc-safety.co.uk	Free advice on diseases in hairdressing
www.hmso.gov.uk	Legislation and regulations
www.tradingstandards.gov.uk	Trading Standards Institute
www.lookfantastic.com	Professional hairdressing products and advice
www.laurandp.co.uk	Educational publications for development of professional hairdressing
www.scott999.fsnet.co.uk	Hairdressing product information
www.nexus.com	Range of hairdressing products
www.tigi.co.uk	Range of hairdressing products
www.schwarzkopf.com	Range of hairdressing products
www.loreal.com	Range of hairdressing products

Magazines and journals

- *Hairdressers Journal*
- *Creative Head*
- *Estetica/Cutting Edge*
- *Black Beauty and Hair*

The evidence from the activities below will cover the Underpinning Knowledge for the Technical Certificate for Advanced Modern Apprenticeships. You will need to take the external test and carry out the practical activities (see City and Guilds Diploma Hairdressing 6915/6913).

ACTIVITY

Outcome 2 Hairdressing, Outcome 3 Barbering

- *State the importance of promoting the benefits of aftercare products and services to the client.*

- *Describe the various steps of the sales process.*

- *Describe what is meant in terms of 'features' and 'benefits' of a product or service.*

- *Describe what is meant by effective communication and explain why this is important.*

- *Describe the features and benefits of the aftercare products and services available within the salon.*

Following the above activities if you are undertaking the Technical Certificate you will need to be assessed on the practical activity pages 20/21 City and Guilds Level 3 Diploma in Hairdressing and/or pages 21, 22, 23 Diploma in Barbering.

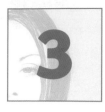

3 | UNIT G9 PROVIDE HAIRDRESSING CONSULTATION SERVICES

1. Identify clients' needs and wishes
2. Analyse the hair, skin and scalp
3. Make recommendations to clients
4. Agree services with your client

CHAPTER CONTENTS

- Consultation
- Self Review
- Types of Consultation
- Avoiding Cross Infection
- Infectious Conditions
- Skin structure
- Structure and Function of the Hair
- Self Review
- Hair and Skin Diseases and Disorders
- Tests for Hair and Skin
- How to Handle Customer Complaints
- Review Questions
- Data Protection Act 1998
- Additional Information
- Activity

Introduction

Consultation and diagnostics is the single most important stage of the hairdressing service. The aim of consultation is to find out what the client wants, their needs and any problems they may have, then to carry out the service to their satisfaction so that they go away happy to pay the bill and return for further treatments. When clients enter the salon they will expect you to be able to help, advise or refer them to a service they require. It may also be necessary to advise them of a service they might not have thought about.

There are various stages in a consultation. The first might be to introduce yourself and the last to go to the basin and shampoo the client's hair. Note down what you think are the other stages in the consultation process. You should be able to mention five other stages. Responses could include:

1. Discuss the client's needs and obtain information.
2. Examine the client's hair and scalp.
3. Explain your findings.
4. Offer a course of action/treatment advice.
5. Decide and confirm with the client the course of treatment to be followed.

This unit will help you to:

- define the meaning of consultation and diagnostics
- identify the needs for consultation and diagnostics
- prepare yourself before a consultation
- plan a consultation
- identify what information to obtain through consultation.

Before starting carry out the following;

1 Write down what you think consultation means.

2 Write down what you think diagnosing means.

Consultation

Before hairdressers can do anything to a client's hair, and before they can get involved in any hairdressing process (e.g. cutting, styling, perming, colouring, etc.), they must have some background knowledge of the client. Consultation and diagnostics are the first steps to take before any of the hairdressing processes.

> **Consultation:** seeking advice or information from a person.
>
> **Diagnostic:** identification of a disease or condition from its signs or symptoms.

The need for consultation and diagnostics in hairdressing is to make sure the treatment chosen for the client is:

- safe (causes no damage to the client or their hair)
- appropriate (suits the client's needs and looks the part)
- effective (the desired result is achieved).

Every client, whether old or new, should have a consultation with the stylist before any treatment begins. By talking to the client you will find out important information which affects the choice of treatment and how it is carried out.

Consultation will:

- find out personal information, i.e. approximate age, lifestyle, and address
- note client's physical characteristics, e.g. face shape, skin colour, build
- find out personal preferences e.g. favourite colours, preferred hair style.

Diagnostics involves identifying:

- client's hair type and condition
- scalp condition
- any hair or scalp problems.

Important points to remember:

- Consultation and diagnostics must be carried out **before the client has their hair shampooed.** It is extremely difficult to identify characteristics of the hair and scalp when they are wet.
- Ask politely and courteously for any personal information, e.g. age, previous treatments, etc.
- Use open-ended questions to gather information. These usually include the words why, how when, where, which and require more than a yes or no answer. Use closed questions to gain agreement – yes/no.

- Talk to the client face to face; try to avoid using the mirror.
- Different treatments will involve asking questions relevant to the service about to be carried out on the client. You will also need to research what previous products and services have been used and personal information relating to their hair and scalp, etc.

Listen carefully, as much of the information will be forthcoming provided you can persuade your client to talk freely. Indeed, this stage of the diagnosis is perhaps the most important, for while you only have a short time to consider the head in front of you, its owner will have been living with it for a lifetime!

Be discreet with the information. Do not let everyone hear your discussion, and place the record card safely away.

Consultation can also inform you about the client's hair and scalp and how they care for them. This can also influence the choice of treatment. For example, you may also need to find out:

- How often they shampoo their hair.
- When they last shampooed their hair.
- What sort of shampoo they used.
- If they have a sensitive scalp.
- If they have had any treatment to their hair recently, i.e. colour, perm, etc.
- When they last visited the hairdresser.

Information can also be gathered by observing the client during the consultation, e.g. the hair colour, and the degree of curl.

Self review

What previous experience do you have? Answer the following.

- What technical services are available in your salon including products, equipment and aftercare products?
- Describe how you would recognise a suspected infection and infestation.
- Describe the structure of the hair (cuticle, cortex and medulla).
- Describe the structure of the skin (hair follicle, dermis, sweat gland, blood supply, arrector pili muscle, sebaceous gland, epidermis and hair shaft).

Think of situations where consultation and diagnostics are necessary, for example, hair and scalp disorders, shampooing and conditioning. Responses could include:

- before a chemical process (perming, tinting)
- before styling (cutting, setting, blow drying, etc.)
- in fact, before any process.

The purpose of consultation and diagnostics in hairdressing is to make sure the treatment chosen for the client is:

- safe (causes no damage to the client or their hair)
- effective (suits the client's needs and looks the part)
- appropriate (the desired result is achieved).

Every client whether old or new should, before any treatment begins, have a consultation and diagnostics meeting with the stylist. By talking to the client you will find out important information which affects the choice of treatment and how it will be carried out. What do you think a consultation should find out? Responses could include:

- personal information (age, lifestyle, address)
- personal preferences (preferred hair style, favourite colour)
- Note client physical characteristics, e.g. face shape, skin colour, build, etc.

What should a diagnostics identify? Responses could include:

- client's hair type and condition
- scalp condition
- any hair or scalp problems.

A good hairdresser will develop a number of qualities that will make a good impression on the client, for example a caring approach, a well-planned appointment system, a confident manner. What other qualities and systems should hairdressers have to carry out a good consultation? Responses could include:

- be well dressed
- speak clearly and politely
- ask appropriate questions
- introduce themself by name
- shake the client's hand
- be discreet
- listen to the client
- be tactful, don't smoke, drink or chew in front or the client.

Types of consultation

Basic consultation

- Greet the client, offer them a seat and position yourself correctly for the consultation.
- Explain why you are providing a consultation and what you hope to achieve as the result.
- Ensure effective communication. Use visual aids if available and appropriate.
- Remember to use both verbal and non-verbal types of communication.
- Use consultation sheets to steer the process and record the findings and agreements.
- Take into account any factors that may limit or affect the services and products that may be used on a client.
- Test where necessary to ensure safe practices and client well-being.
- Discreetly check for any hair or scalp disorders.
- Make sure that the client is encouraged to ask about areas of which they are unsure.
- Agreement is made (by client and hairdresser) on course of action.
- Advise client of time and cost.
- Summarise to make sure there is no misunderstanding.
- Offer advice on hair care, styling products and aftercare recommendations.

Advanced consultation

- Listen to client expectations – does the client have something specific in mind? Interpret the client's request.
- Review client's lifestyle – looks required, work aspects, age, fashion needs and client's general activities.

- Observe client's physical features – body size, profile and head shape, prominent facial features, bone structure, skin tone and colour, etc.
- Look at hair constraints – movement and growth patterns, texture, condition, distribution, etc.
- Consider manageability – ease of styling, time available for client to style hair, etc.
- Discuss cost implications.

Shampoo and conditioner consultation

(following on from basic and advanced consultation)

- Analyse hair and scalp for condition.
- Report immediately any sign of abnormality.
- Enquire how frequently the client washes their hair.
- Assess the hair and scalp and choose the shampoo that is most suited for the hair (e.g. coconut for dry hair, citrus for greasy hair, pre-treatment shampoo for perms).
- Assess the condition of hair and decide choice of conditioner (e.g. surface, penetrating).
- Offer advice on which products should be used at home.
- Describe what the pH scale is and explain the average pH values of acid, alkali, neutral, normal hair and scalp, pre-perm shampoo and pH balance shampoo and conditioner.

Cutting and styling consultation

(following on from basic, advanced and shampoo consultation)

- Discuss with client what is required and consider the client's needs.
- Examine the hair type, texture, colour, quality, quantity and access limitations.
- Consider the client's natural direction, movement, growth patterns and whether the hair is curly, wavy or straight.
- Analyse the client's requests and make sure you interpret your client's wishes correctly.
- Agree how much hair should be cut off to make sure there is no misunderstanding.
- Advise the client of time and cost.
- Advise client on a hair maintenance programme.

Colour consultation

(following on from basic and advance consultation)

- Refer to client's record card, if available.
- Analyse the hair's condition, porosity, elasticity and texture.
- Examine the hair for previous chemical treatments.
- Identify the natural base colour of the hair.
- Note the percentage of white hair present.
- If necessary conduct colour tests (e.g. porosity, skin, test cutting) and record the result.
- Decide on what sort of colouring to carry out and agree with the client on what product to use. Use the colour chart for the client and hairdresser agreement.
- Summarise to make sure there is no misunderstanding.
- Advise on how long the process will take and how much it will cost.

Perm consultation

(following on from basic and advanced consultation)

- Refer to the client's record card, if available.
- Discuss the client's requirements and expectations from the perm.
- Examine the hair and scalp.
- Examine the hair for previous chemical treatments.
- Consider the client's cut and style.
- Analyse the hair texture and carry out any necessary tests (e.g. porosity, test curl, incompatibility).
- Consider the type of curl needed, winding technique required and product to be used.
- Summarise to make sure there is no misunderstanding.
- Advise client of time and cost.

Dressing hair consultation

(following on from basic, advanced and shampoo consultation)

- Discuss the client's requirements and wishes.
- Consider the client's cut, natural direction, movement and growth patterns of hair and whether it is curly, wavy or straight.
- Discuss with the client any application of aids to drying and shaping (e.g. gel, setting lotion).
- Summarise to make sure there is no misunderstanding.
- Explain the importance of continuous consultation throughout the hairdressing service.
- Advise the client on time and cost.
- Advise client on any aftercare products and give advice on how client can achieve a similar style at home.

> *Remember: Consultation should involve making suggestions and offering expert advice on a hairstyle to suit the client's appearance and lifestyle, diagnosing hair or scalp conditions. All consultations should be carried out before a service begins, when the hair is still dry.*

The consultation process

1. Client enters the salon.
2. Client is greeted and offered a seat.
3. Client is given a consultation by the hairdresser.
4. Any necessary tests are done and a check is made for infectious conditions.
5. Agreement is made (by client and hairdresser) on the course of action.
6. Service is given.

Avoiding cross infection

Germs and bacteria are on our hands, in our noses and mouths – basically everywhere. These are called micro-organisms and are harmful bacteria. This is why it is imperative that you should sterilise all tools and equipment between each client, to minimise cross infection.

Infections can be spread very easily in the salon by the following means:

- dirty tools and equipment

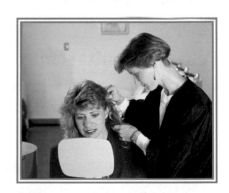

Figure 3.1 Analysing a client's hair physiology

- haircuttings on the floor
- unwashed gowns and towels
- not washing your hands after using the toilet
- bad personal hygiene
- coughing and sneezing over clients
- dirty salon.

Germs and bacteria spread easily in warm, moist, damp conditions. Barbers and hairdressers may come into contact with clients who have viruses and infections that can be spread by touching the hair and skin. The spread of infection can be reduced by recommending that the client's hair is shampooed prior to services and that tools and equipment are sterilised after use on each client.

Sterilisation

Sterilisation is the complete destruction of all living organisms on an object. The three main forms of sterilisation used in salons are heat, radiation and chemical. More information is included within Unit G1.

Infectious conditions

Infections and infestation

Infections are caused by harmful germs and bacteria. These include colds and flu, conjunctivitis, ringworm, cold sores, impetigo, boils and warts. Infestations are caused by animal parasites living on the human body, such as head lice and scabies caused by the itch mite. All hairdressers and barbers must be able to recognise the symptoms of these conditions and be able to tell if they are infectious or non-infectious.

Infections are infectious and can be spread from person to person indirectly through the air or water, for example the cold and flu virus. Transmission can occur through ingestion, direct contact, indirect contact, droplets and body fluids. They are also contagious and can be passed from person to person by direct contact and by contaminated tools and equipment such as towels, brushes and combs in the salon.

Bacteria

These organisms need warmth and moisture to multiply quickly in or outside the body. Bacterial infections, such as boils and impetigo, are treated with antibiotics.

Fungal

A plant form or parasite that feeds on the keratin (protein) of skin, for example ringworm and athlete's foot. They grow and multiply in similar conditions to bacteria.

Virus

Viruses survive in the living cells of the human body, but once outside the body they die. These include colds, flu and even HIV (AIDS). Most viral infections can be treated with antibiotics.

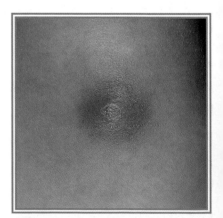

Figure 3.2 Bacterial infection

Parasite

Parasites are classed as infestations as they involve animal parasites. Head lice and scabies live on the human body. These parasites need nourishment from the host to survive – they pierce the skin to take blood in order to reproduce and multiply.

An infestation can develop into a secondary infection such as impetigo, because the infestation has caused itching and breaking of the skin, allowing the bacteria to enter.

Disorders of the hair

None of the following conditions are contagious.

Canities

Canities is the technical term for grey hair. Its immediate cause is the loss of natural pigment in the hair. There are two types:

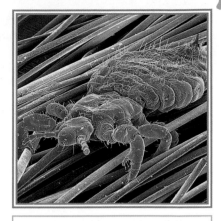

Figure 3.4 Head lice

- Congenital canities exists at or before birth. It occurs in albinos and occasionally in persons with normal hair. A patchy type of congenital canities may develop either slowly or rapidly depending upon the cause of the condition.

- Acquired canities may be due to old age, or onset may occur prematurely in early adult life. Causes of acquired canities may be worry, anxiety, nervous strain, prolonged illness or heredity.

Ringed hair

Ringed hair has alternate bands of white and dark hair.

Hypertrichosis

Hypertrichosis or *hirsuties* means superfluous hair, an abnormal development of hair on areas of the body normally bearing only downy hair. Treatment: Tweeze or remove by depilatories, electrolysis, shaving or epilation.

Trichoptilosis

Trichoptilosis (see Figure 3.19) is the technical term for split ends. Treatment: The hair should be well-oiled to soften and lubricate the dry ends. The splits must be removed by cutting. Split ends may be temporarily treated by proprietary brands of split-end treatments, but these are purely temporary.

Trichorrexis nodosa

Trichorrexis nodosa or *knotted hair* (see Figure 3.20), is a dry, brittle condition including the formation of nodular swellings along the hair shaft. The hair breaks easily and there is a brush-like spreading out of the fibres of the broken-off hair along the hair shaft. Softening the hair with conditioners may prove beneficial.

Monilethrix

Monilethrix is the technical term for beaded hair. The hair breaks between the beads or nodes. Scalp and hair treatments may improve the hair condition.

Fragilitas crinium

Fragilitas crinium is the technical term for brittle hair, or split ends. The hairs may split at any part of their length. Conditioning hair treatment may be recommended, most effective is to cut and remove the split.

Disorders of the scalp

Just as the skin is continually being shed and replaced, the uppermost layer of the scalp is also being cast off all the time. Ordinarily, these horny scales loosen and fall off freely. The natural shedding of these horny scales should not be mistaken for dandruff.

Dandruff

Dandruff consists of small, white scales that usually appear on the scalp and hair. The medical term for dandruff is *pityriasis*. Long neglected, excessive dandruff can lead to baldness. The nature of dandruff is not clearly defined by medical authorities although it is generally believed to be of infectious origin. Some authorities hold that it is due to a specific microbe.

A direct cause of dandruff is the excessive shedding of the epithelial, or surface cells. Instead of growing to the surface and falling off, these horny scales accumulate on the scalp.

Indirect or associated causes of dandruff are a sluggish condition of the scalp, possibly due to poor circulation, infection, injury, lack of nerve stimulation, improper diet and uncleanliness. Contributing causes are the use of strong shampoos and insufficient rinsing of the hair after shampooing. The two principal types of dandruff are:

● Pityriasis capitis simplex – dry type (see Figure 3.4).
● Pityriasis steatoides – a greasy or waxy type (see Figure 3.5).

Pityriasis capitis simplex (dandruff) is characterised by an itchy scalp and small white scales, which are usually attached to the scalp in masses, or scattered loosely in the hair. Occasionally, they are so profuse that they fall to the shoulders. Dry dandruff is often the result of a sluggish scalp caused by poor circulation, lack of nerve stimulation, improper diet, emotional and glandular disturbances, or uncleanliness. Treatment: Frequent scalp treatments, use of mild shampoos, regular scalp massage, daily use of antiseptic scalp lotions, and applications of scalp ointments.

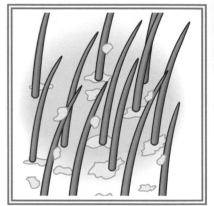

Figure 3.4 Pityriasis capitis simplex (dandruff)

Pityriasis steatoides (greasy or waxy type of dandruff) is a scaly condition of the epidermis (surface skin). The scales become mixed with sebum, causing them to stick to the scalp in patches. There may be itchiness, causing the person to scratch the scalp. If the greasy scales are torn off, bleeding or oozing of sebum may follow. Medical treatment is advisable. Both forms of dandruff are considered to be contagious and can be spread by the common use of brushes, combs and other articles. Therefore, the hairdresser must take the necessary precautions to sterilise everything that comes into contact with the client.

Alopecia

Alopecia is the technical term for any abnormal hair loss. The natural falling out of the hair should not be confused with alopecia. When hair has gone through its growing stage (Anagen), it falls out and is replaced by a new hair. The natural shedding of hair occurs most frequently in spring and autumn. Hair loss due to alopecia is not replaced unless special treatments are given to encourage hair loss. Hairstyles such as ponytails and tight braids cause tension on the hair and can contribute to constant hair loss or baldness.

Alopecia senilis is the form of baldness that occurs in old age. This loss of hair is permanent. It is not contagious.

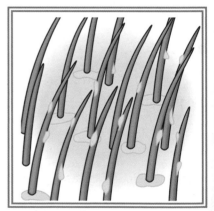

Figure 3.5 Pityriasis steatoides (greasy dandruff)

Alopecia prematura is the form of baldness that begins any time before middle age with a slow, thinning process. This condition is caused when hairs fall out and are replaced by weaker ones. It is not contagious.

Alopecia areata is the sudden falling out of hair in round patches, or baldness in spots, sometimes caused by anaemia, scarlet fever, typhoid fever or syphilis. Patches are round or irregular in shape and can vary in size from 1.25 to 5 or 7.5 cm ($\frac{1}{2}$" to 2" or 3") in diameter. Affected areas are slightly depressed, smooth and very pale due to a decreased blood supply. In most conditions of alopecia areata, the nervous system has been subjected to some injury. Since the flow of blood is influenced by the nervous system, the affected area is also poorly nourished (see Figure 3.6).

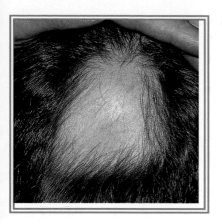

Figure 3.6 Alopecia areata

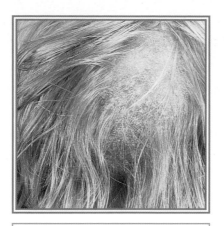

Figure 3.7 Tinea capitis

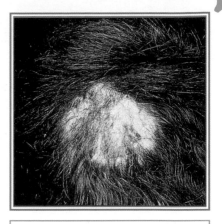

Figure 3.8 Tinea favosa (honeycomb ringworm)

Treatment for alopecia

Alopecia appears in a variety of different forms, caused by many abnormal conditions. Sometimes an alopecia condition can be improved by proper scalp treatments.

Control of Substances Hazardous to Health (COSHH) Regulations 1999

The law requires employers to control exposure to hazardous substances to prevent ill health. Using chemicals or other hazardous substances in the hairdresser's and barber's can put people's health at risk. Employers have to protect both employees and others who may be exposed to hazardous substances by complying with the Regulations. You need to assess the risks and take any measures needed to control exposure and establish good working practices. More information and guidance is provided in Unit G1.

Skin structure

The skin has two main structures:

1 The dermis – or true skin – where all the organs of the skin are.

2 The epidermis, the part of the skin that we see. The epidermis also has various layers: stratum germinativum, stratum spinosum, stratum granulosum, stratum lucidum, stratum corneum

Under the skin is subcutaneous tissue. Important structures that support the skin are:

● The hair follicle and its structure – the hair is formed and grows from the follicle

● The sebaceous oil gland – lubricates and helps protect the skin secreted into the follicle

● The arrector pili muscle – causes goose bumps on the skin; helps to regulate the body's temperature

● The sudoriferous or sweat gland – excretes waste products and secretes sweat on to the skin, which helps to regulate body temperature

● The blood supply – nerves and their endings – giving sensations of touch, heat, cold and pain. The dermis is well supplied with blood vessels; partly to supply nutrients and oxygen to the various glands, to allow the skin to play its part in regulating body temperature and to carry away de-oxygenated blood and waste products.

Growth and structure of the hair

At the base of each hair follicle (the tube-like depression in the skin through which the hair grows) is a living hair bulb. This bulb is composed of cells that rapidly divide to produce the components of hair fibre. Through this division, these

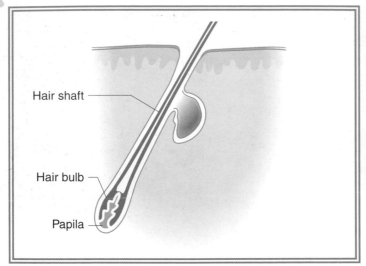

Hair shaft

Hair bulb

Papila

Figure 3.9 The hair follicle

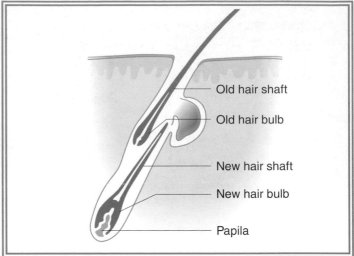

Old hair shaft

Old hair bulb

New hair shaft

New hair bulb

Papila

Figure 3.10 New hair growing in follicle

cells are forced up the follicle. At the same time they are changing shape, losing moisture and becoming joined together by a system of cross linkages, and suffer the loss of their nuclei by enzyme action leading to the death of the cell. *Keratinisation* is the name given to this hardening process, which takes place on top and just above the hair bulb. These cells are made up of proteins collectively known as *keratin*, with additional small amounts of carbohydrates, oils and minerals (approximately 6%).

Among the cells of the upper part of the papilla are *melanocytes*, which distribute minute granules of the hair's natural pigments called *melanin* and *pheo-melanin*. These are almost entirely found in the cortex. With age, or sometimes as a result of hair regrowth (after alopecia areata, for example), hair grows with no pigmentation, a condition called *canities* (white hair).

Whilst in the follicle the hair is surrounded by the root sheath which interlocks with the cuticle of the hair to grow at the same rate. The root sheath breaks down at the level of the sebaceous glands. The passage of the hair further up the follicle is eased by the presence of sebum.

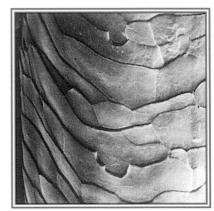

Figure 3.11 Magnified view of hair cuticle, which is composed of keratin

The hair grows out of the head in different directions. It is important to look for these growth patterns for cutting and styling the hair.

It is the angle at which the follicles lie and their distribution (or pattern) on the scalp that produces the natural direction of the hair growth and produces the natural partings. The natural wave pattern of a person's hair is inherited from their parents, as is their colour.

Hair texture is described by how fine, coarse or medium textured the hair is. It is the diameter of the hair not the amount of hair on the head (abundance) that determines hair texture.

Fine hair has very close, compact cuticles, therefore is generally resistant to certain products or treatments.

Coarse hair has more raised, lifted cuticles, therefore is less resistant to products or treatments.

You can feel the texture of the hair by running the thumb and finger along the length of the hair from the root top point. Fine hair is small in diameter and feels smooth and silky along its length. Coarse hair, because of the way it is formed, has larger diameter, the cuticle is slightly raised and it feels rough to the touch.

Knowledge and practice at identifying hair texture helps with the selection of the right product and the hair treatment to be used. Many products that are used in the salon need to be selected to suit the hair type or texture.

The amount of curl, wave and straightness of the hair affects its texture by giving the hair more or less volume. Perming can improve hair texture.

At one time it was thought that the shape of the follicle determined the natural wave or curliness of the hair. However, recent evidence suggests that the natural curl formation takes place in the dermal papilla or hair bulb when the cell division around the diameter of the hair is uneven. This causes hair to bend resulting in wavy or curly hair.

Condition of the hair can change its texture because the cuticle could be raised, thickening the diameter of the hair. Care must be taken when giving treatments to clients to limit damage to the cuticle. It must not be damaged to the extent that the hair becomes difficult to manage and looks dull, dry and lifeless.

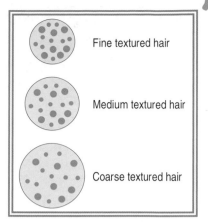

Figure 3.12 Relative diameters of various hair strands (shown enlarged)

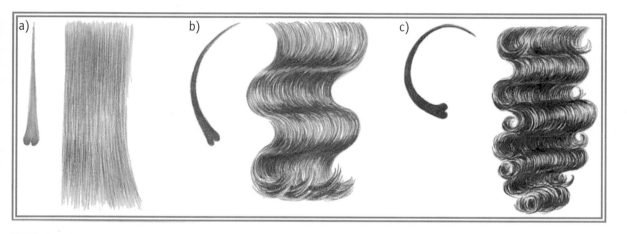

Figure 3.13 a Straight hair; b Wavy hair; c Curly hair

According to its texture, the hair has a diameter of between 1/500th of an inch and 1/1500th of and inch. The average area of a head is approximately 120 sq. inches, with approximately 1000 hairs growing on each square inch. The number of hairs on the head varies between 100,000 for a very dark head of hair (in Caucasians; usually the darker the colour, the coarser the texture) to 140,000 for a head of light blond hair.

Hair grows at about 1.25 cm or $\frac{1}{2}$ inch per month due to cell division down at the hair root. There are about 120,000 hairs on a full scalp of hair, and any one of these hairs lasts on the head from one to seven years. During its life expectancy the hair passes through the three stages of the hair growth cycle.

Growth cycle (anagen, catagen, telogen)

Protein is necessary for the healthy growth of our bodies and also for healthy hair growth. In fact, good hair conditions with a healthy diet, one that contains plenty of protein, such as fish, meat, eggs, cheese, etc. A diet lacking in protein will not only affect the hair's condition but will also slow down its growth. Other physical factors that can affect hair growth include health, age, nutrition, shock, hormones, pregnancy, genetics, ethnicity, and forms of alopecia.

About 100 scalp hairs a day are normally lost and replaced by new hairs in the *Anagen* stage. The common forms of baldness are caused by the lack of new hairs being produced. For various reasons, follicles cease hair production. Baldness of various kinds is technically called alopecia.

Anagen is the active growing stage and lasts between two and six years. Approximately 80% to 90% of all hairs on a healthy scalp are in the anagen phase at any given time.

The second stage is a transitional one known as the *Catagen* phase. The activity of the hair bulb slows down, producing fewer and fewer new cells, until it ceases altogether. At any given time, approximately 1% to 2% of all hairs on the scalp are in the catagen phase.

The *Telogen* stage is the final one, where the bulb has a resting period which lasts for three to four months. During, this stage, the hair is released from the follicle and by the end of this period new hair has started to grow from the papilla.

Structure and function of the hair

To be able to perform treatments and services for clients as well as being able to identify hair problems, you need to have an understanding of the material that hairdressers work with.

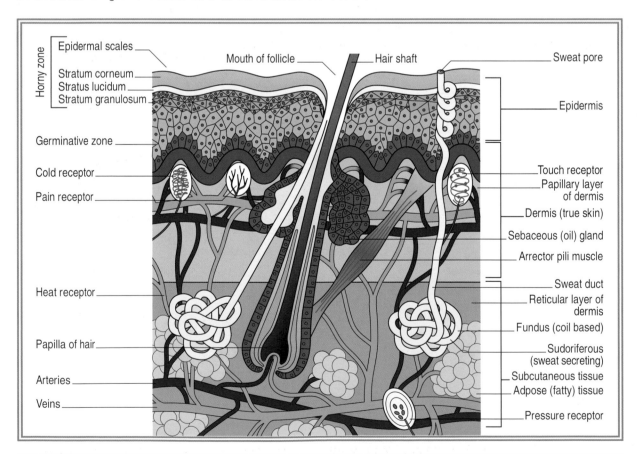

Figure 3.14 A cross section of the scalp

Different hair types:

- Caucasian (European)
- Negroid (Afro/Caribbean)
- Mongoloid (Asian).

The various types of hair found on the body:

- vellus hair (fine, short, fluffy hair which covers most parts of the body. It can be seen clearly on the faces of women)
- terminal hair (longer, coarser hair found on the head, on the chest, and in the pubic region)
- lanugo hair (fine, downy hair that covers the body of the unborn child: it is lost just before or around birth).

There are three layers that make up the basic structure of the hair:

- the **cuticle** (the outer layer)
- the **cortex** (the middle layer that makes the bulk of the hair)
- the **medulla** (the centre core, which is sometimes missing in very fine hair).

The purpose of the outer layer, the **cuticle** is to:

- protect (the structure of the hair)
- regulate (liquids entering the hair structure)
- hold the hair together.

The bulk of the hair is made up of the hair's cortex (the middle layer of the hair). It consists of bundles of cortical fibres twisting around each other and surrounded by a putty-like, filler substance.

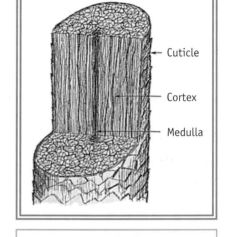

Figure 3.15 Structure of a hair

The hair is formed from five basic chemical elements: carbon (50%), oxygen, nitrogen, hydrogen and sulphur. These elements form amino acids, which form polypeptides, which form proteins.

Bundles of polypeptide chains wrap around each other to form larger groups of hair fibres that are surrounded by the filler (the matrix).

- Polypeptide chain
- Microfibril
- Macrofibril
- Cortical fibril

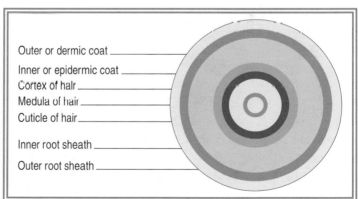

Figure 3.16 Cross-section of the hair and follicle

The cuticle layer, which protects this inner structure of the hair, is several layers thick and lays from root to tip.

Hair is acidic and has a pH scale of 4.5.–5.5. It is very important that we keep the hair's natural acidity as this keeps the hair in a good condition and enables the hair to stretch and return into its natural shape.

When setting and blow-drying, hair changes from alpha to beta-keratin as it is stretched and dried into its new position. Hair can stretch up to 30% when wet depending on its elasticity.

As hairdressers it is important to know the pH chart, as we are dealing with chemicals and hairdressing products.

- Hair has a natural pH of 4.5.–5.5
- Shampoos and conditioners can help to control the hair's natural pH if used correctly
- 1–6.9 is Acid. This reads red if using litmus paper to test for acidity.
- 7 is Neutral. This will read green showing that it is neutral.
- 7.1–14 is Alkali. This will read blue on the litmus paper showing alkalinity.

If we use too strong an acid or too strong an alkali on hair then it can start to become porous, weakening the hair structure and it may even disintegrate. These will remove the acid mantle, which coats the hair, which is a combination of sebum and sweat (salt and water).

The acid mantle is the body's first defence against bacteria as it provides a waterproof coating to protect the hair and skin. If this is removed the skin and hair will become porous and may crack or split leaving it open to bacteria.

Always use pH-balanced shampoos and conditioners to restore the hair back to its natural acidity especially after chemical treatments.

Hair chemistry

Proteins: simple and complex proteins, amino acids, polypeptides (disulphide bonds, hydrogen bonds, salt bonds).

Keratin protein: soft and hard keratin, alpha [α] and beta [β] keratin

pH scale: acid, neutral, alkaline

Hair is **hygroscopic**, in other words it is able to absorb moisture from the atmosphere. Depending on conditions of humidity, the hair can hold up to 15% or more of its total weight in water. Warmth can increase the hair's ability to absorb moisture.

Hair is **elastic**. The ability of the hair to stretch and return to its original length allows hairdressers to style the hair using dryers, brushes or rollers, etc, by changing the position of the weaker bonds in the cortex.

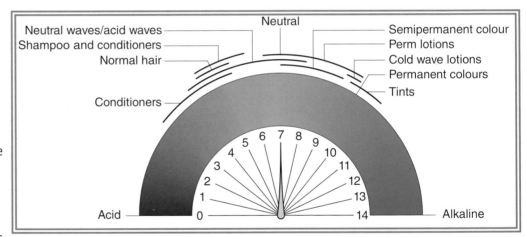

Figure 3.17 Relative pH of hairdressing substances

The ability of the hair to change its structure allows us to colour, permanently curl and straighten. Strong chemicals such as perm lotion and permanent hair colouring will damage the hair. Hair should never be over processed (lotions left on too long, the wrong type of product or strength used, even poorly formulated shampoo will damage hair).

Harsh physical treatment with heat, hair bands, hair pins and grips, hair extensions, twiddling the hair, etc, will damage temporarily and could even damage the hair permanently.

The environment: pollution, sun, salt water and swimming pool water all damage hair.

Hair looks best when it is in good condition. Exactly what 'good condition' means is difficult to define, but it does involve factors such as:

- manageability
- good shine

- pliability and elasticity

- soft to the touch and has 'body'.

The hair shaft is dead and cannot repair itself in the way that living parts of the body can. Yet the condition of the individual hair shaft determines the overall condition of the whole head of hair.

In the average life of a typical scalp hair, it may have been:

- brushed and combed nearly 10,000 times

- washed (using a shampoo) about 600 times

- permanently waved about 16 times

- tinted (perhaps with a bleach included) 40 times.

It says much for the toughness of the hair structure that it can stand up to all this punishment without disintegrating. Hair does 'age', however, and the oldest hair is that at the hair points, which has usually suffered more damage than that near the scalp. This needs to be considered in terms of the processing time in bleaching, tinting and perming hair.

A key factor of hair condition is the degree of cuticle damage. This can result from a number of factors which we discuss when we start to look at hair conditioning.

Self review

- Name the substance the hair is made from and explain the structure of the hair, how the hair grows and how natural hair colour is formed.

- List the properties of the hair, what damages it and how you can repair it.

A thorough knowledge of the hair is also required:

- Know how hair is affected by shampoo and conditioners used.

- Be able to inform clients what is happening to their hair during various processes.

- Know what hair in good condition looks and feels like.

- Know how hair is affected by the way you treat it.

- Know how to treat hair properly.

Name the parts of the skin and hair

- The hair shaft

- The hair root

- The hair bulb

- The hair follicle

- The root sheath

- The dermis

- The epidermis

- The subcutaneous (fatty) layer

- The sweat (suderoferous) gland

- The sweat pore (duct)

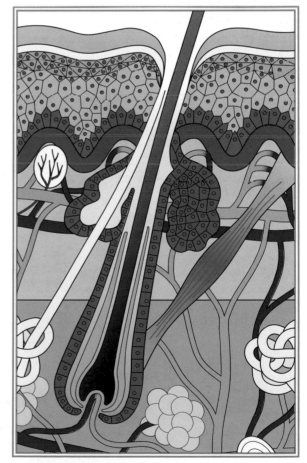

Figure 3.18 Cross-section of skin and hair

- The oil (sebaceous) gland
- The arrector pili muscle
- The papilla
- The blood capillaries
- The nerve endings
- The cuticle
- The cortex
- The medulla

Hair and skin diseases and disorders

To perform hairdressing services safely and professionally you need to be able to identify hair and skin disorders and diseases. You will need to be able to:

- list the basic structure of the hair and skin
- state the difference between contagious and non-contagious diseases
- list non-contagious hair and skin disorders
- list contagious hair and skin disorders.

As a hairdresser, what do you think are the most common problems that clients have with their hair and scalp? Responses could include:

- greasy hair and scalp
- dry hair and scalp
- itchy, sensitive scalp

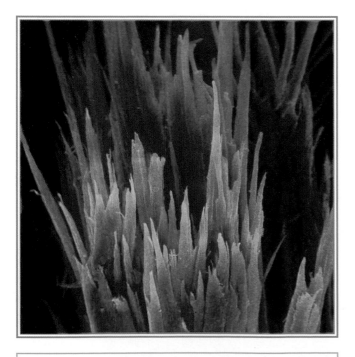

Figure 3.19 Trichoptilosis

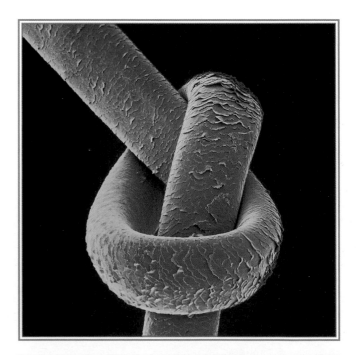

Figure 3.20 Trichorexis nodosa

- dandruff, psoriasis

- split ends

- damaged hair through the environment or hair treatments

- dull, limp, frizzy hair

- baldness

- ringworm, impetigo, head lice.

There are a number of hair and scalp problems that hairdressers have to deal with. Firstly we will deal with scalp problems, but before we can do that we need a basic understanding of the skin structure. What do you think is the function or purpose of the skin? Responses should include:

- it helps regulate body temperature

- it secretes – oil to lubricate the skin

- it excretes – sweat and waste products

- it allows us to feel sensations – heat, cold, pain and touch.

Sometimes the skin does not function correctly or it becomes infected and shows symptoms of the problem. For instance, dandruff is recognised by flakes of skin on the shoulders and dry, scaling scalp.

Can you name some common disorders that hairdressers may come across? We'll start with dandruff. Responses should include: greasy skin, dry skin, psoriasis, eczema/dermatitis, warts (verrucae), herpes (cold sore, shingles), impetigo, ring worm (tinea capitis), folliculitus, furunculosis (boils and abscesses), sycosis, acne, head lice (pediculosis capitas).

Some of these diseases and problems are infectious (they can be passed on to another person), and must always be treated by a general practitioner (doctor), a health visitor or with specialist advice. Non-infectious conditions can often be treated by the hairdresser.

It is suggested that a detailed study of each disorder is made, starting with those that are treated only by a medical practitioner, before moving on to those that can be treated in the salon. The cause and symptom of each disorder must be covered.

Disorders that must be treated only by a medical practitioner, a health visitor or with specialist advice are:

- impetigo

- tinea capitis (see Fig 3.8)

- pediculosis capitis (see Fig 3.4).

Tests for hair and skin

Porosity test

This checks the cuticle for condition, damage and being open.

The test is used when determining the choice and selection of chemicals or treatments to the hair. The porosity of the hair can vary along its length as well as in different areas of the head, so a careful check of the whole head should be carried out.

Draw the hair strand between the fingers, points to roots. Any resistance to this movement indicates the cuticle is raised and the hair is porous.

This test is used before permanent waving, colouring or bleaching and before straightening or relaxing.

Elasticity test

This is used to determine the strength of the hair. It is used before permanent waving, colouring or bleaching and before straightening or relaxing. Hair should stretch approximately 30% to 50% of its length and return to its original length. If it stretches and breaks easily the hair needs to be internally conditioned with a restructurant.

Grasp the hair near to the points and hold firmly while pulling at the points. Hair with a low level of elasticity will break easily.

Incompatibility test

This test is used to determine whether hair has been treated with an incompatible chemical (metal based).

It is used before permanent waving, colouring or bleaching and before straightening or relaxing. Take a test cutting of hair and immerse this in a solution of hydrogen peroxide to which a few drops of perm lotion has been added. Vigorous bubbling, discoloration, heat generation, and eventual hair disintegration indicate the presence of metallic slats on the hair. This hair should not receive any chemical processes that involve oxidisation.

Test cutting

This is a sample of hair taken from the head to determine what has happened before or to see if the right result can be achieved, without affecting other hair on the head. The best way to take a test cutting is to section a piece of hair to one side of the occipital bone at the back of the head. Back comb the section, then slither cut the hair off. Using this technique allows you to take hair without a missing piece being noticeable.

Strand test

This is used to follow colour development during tinting or bleaching at the hair root and/or along its length. Product is wiped from the hair strand so that the emerging colour effect can be viewed. Remember that when moist the hair colour will often appear slightly darker than when dry.

Test curl

This is used to check that the correct rod size and lotion is used when perming, and to find out the processing time.

It is used before permanent waving and consists of winding and processing sections of hair using differing size curlers and/or strengths of perm lotion to determine which will most effectively produce the result required. The term is often also used to check the development of a permanent wave by partially unwinding a curler.

Skin test (allergy)

This test is used to find out whether a person is allergic to a product and is usually associated with para-dye and reactions to the tint.

It is used before every permanent para-dye colour application. A small amount of the product is applied to a cleaned pulse point, usually behind the client's ear or in the crook of the elbow. The product is left for 24 hours to determine whether any reaction occurs. If a reaction does occur it must be assumed unsafe to proceed with an oxidation tint with the client.

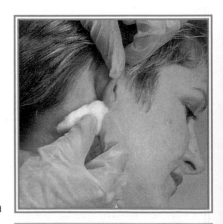

Figure 3.21 Clean patch test area

How to handle customer complaints

Complaints should be responded to promptly and positively on all occasions. Whether a complaint is well founded or not is irrelevant. If the client perceives that there is something wrong, this perception must be managed. It is in the salon's interests to ensure that clients are satisfied with the service they receive. A dissatisfied client can provide adverse impressions to other clients and potential clients. Pointers to good practice include:

- Acknowledge the customer. Make eye contact and ask the customer the nature of the problem.

- Take them to a quiet place and discuss the problem while seated.

- Listen to what they have to say. Body language is important. Face them and look interested. It is in your interest to fully understand the true nature of the client's concerns. You may have to ask further questions to gather sufficient information to be able to offer effective advice and solutions.

- To show you are listening you could make notes, say 'yes' or nod, show empathy and concern that your client feels they have a complaint and the distress this is causing.

- Mirror their actions.

- Sympathise and apologise.

- Then, if necessary, inform your superior and let them take care of the troubled customer.

- If the customer can be handled without informing your superior then:

  ▶ Summarise and clarify the issue.

  ▶ If there has been a fault in the service provided, suggest an alternative for action. Do not look to apportion blame but look forward to the remedy.

  ▶ Whenever possible gain client agreement.

  ▶ Make a record of the issue and subsequent agreements.

Remember:
- *Always be polite to the client.*
- *Be positive.*
- *Stay calm at all times.*
- *Genuine and valid customer complaints should serve as development points, so consider what future actions are necessary to avoid similar situations occurring again.*

Never

- Talk to the dissatisfied client in a busy place.

- Shout or raise your voice at the client.

- Interrupt the client at any time.

- Argue with the client.

- Personally take the blame for the problem.

- NEVER swear at, or use offensive or abusive language towards, the client!

Review Questions

1 Design a consultation sheet that takes into consideration services available e.g. shampooing and conditioning, cutting, styling, colouring, perming, shaving, massage, etc.

2 When carrying out consultations what information would you need for a colour service that you would not need for a cutting service?

3 In a consultation what information would you need for all services?

4 Why is it important to carry out a consultation prior to shampooing a client's hair and scalp?

5 What would you do if your client had a contagious disease?

continued...

...continued

Review Questions

6 What are your responsibilities regarding the handling of client information with regard to the Data Protection Act?

7 Why is it important to keep up to date with current and emerging trends?

8 Why is it important to carry out hair and skin tests?

9 Why is it important to listen to the client and record information?

10 Why is it important to recommend the correct products?

11 Why is it important to follow manufacturer's information?

12 What are your legal responsibilities for reporting infectious diseases?

Data Protection Act 1998

This Act requires all organisations that hold data and personal information about living people to register with the Information Commissioner.

The Act requires that data held by organisations should be:

- fairly and lawfully processed
- processed for limited purposes
- adequate, relevant and not excessive
- accurate
- not kept longer than necessary
- processed in accordance with the data subject's rights
- secure
- not transferred to countries without adequate protection.

Within the salon data may be held about clients, staff and potential staff (job applicants). Whether kept electronically or in paper files this data must be stored securely and its contents communicated only to authorised people. The salon determines those authorised and will include this information in their registration with the Commissioner. The commission provides guidelines in acceptable practice. Those providing data must give their consent for its intended use. Each organisation should have a person responsible (Compliance Manager) for overseeing the collection, storage and processing of data and in ensuring that all staff are aware of their responsibilities for this.

Additional information

Useful websites

Website Addresses	Content
www.habia.org.uk	Hairdressing and Beauty Industry Authority. Downloads available including references to other websites
www.bbc-safety.co.uk	Free advice on diseases in hairdressing
www.hse.org.uk	Information commissioner
www.lookfantastic.com	Professional hairdressing products and advice
www.laurandp.co.uk	Educational publications for development of professional hairdressing
www.scott999.fsnet.co.uk	Hairdressing product information
www.keratin.com	Hair and scalp disorders
www.trichologists.org.uk	Institute of Trichologists

The evidence from the activities below will cover the Underpinning Knowledge for the Technical Certificate for Advanced Modern Apprenticeships. You will need to take the external test and carry out the practical activities. (See City and Guilds Diploma Hairdressing 6915/6913.)

ACTIVITY

Outcome 1

• State why it is important to identify factors that may limit, affect or prohibit the services and products that can be used. Factors: adverse conditions (hair, skin or scalp), incompatibility of previous service or products used, head and face shape, hair growth pattern, client image, client wishes, lifestyle.

• Recognise adverse hair, skin and scalp conditions and describe the action that should be taken when providing a service in the salon.

• Describe the various types of tests that are carried out for different services.

• Recognise suspected infections and infestations and describe the action that should be taken by the salon if their presence is suspected. Infections: bacterial, viral, fungal; Infestations: animal parasites.

• Describe the structure of the hair and skin. Range: epidermis, dermis, sweat gland, erector pili muscle, blood capillaries, hair bulb, hair shaft, follicle, dermal papilla.

• Briefly describe the difference in the hair structure between different ethnic hair types.

• Explain how to provide advice to clients in a way that will maintain client goodwill and confidentiality. State why this is important.

Following the above activities, if you are undertaking the Technical Certificate you will need to be assessed on the practical activity pages 25, 26 of City and Guilds Level 3 Diploma in Hairdressing and/or pages 26 Diploma Barbering.

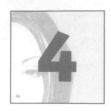

4 UNIT G10 SUPPORT CUSTOMER SERVICE IMPROVEMENTS

1 Use feedback to identify potential customer service improvements

2 Contribute to the implementation of changes in customer service

3 Assist with the evaluation of changes in customer services

CHAPTER CONTENTS

- *What is Customer Service?*
- *Gaining Customer Feedback*
- *Improving Customer Service*
- *Reporting Changes within the Client Services*
- *Review Questions*

What is customer service?

In this unit we will look at the whole experience of the client from the time they make contact, enter the salon and continue with the home maintenance programme. We will evaluate strategies by collecting evidence that can be appropriate to improving customer services. By this we mean looking at volume of sales, new and repeat business, customer awareness, etc. So what type of service do you give to your clients and how do you rate the level of that service? We know the client wants a good hairstyle but they also come to the salon for a number of other reasons, for example, advice and guidance, relaxing atmosphere, and because it has a good reputation. These reasons are important as you can start measuring the level of success by the amount of repeat business and increase in product and customer sales.

If the client enjoys the experience then they are more likely to return, thus building up customer loyalty, which will increase repeat business and ultimately lead to your ability to earn more money. However, it is not just about earning money; it is also about making people look and feel good and gaining job satisfaction.

The customer service package varies from salon to salon and it is worthwhile finding out how your competitors are performing and what they have to offer. The level of service you provide will be one factor that influences the price you charge. Some clients have more disposable income than others therefore you need to be sensitive to their needs.

Gaining customer feedback

So why does the client come to you? You need to find this out to see how you are performing and to action any weaknesses. Below is a sample questionnaire which you might find useful as a starting point if you do not have one already.

By collecting this information you can then start to summarise the information and evaluate it and action any weak points. It is important to discuss the results with team as everyone has a vital role to play, e.g. receptionist, technician assistant, etc. The questionnaire needs to be quick and easy to use. By offering an incentive for filling it in straight away you are more likely to get the client to complete the questionnaire.

CLIENT SATISFACTION SURVEY

SAMPLE

We are constantly trying to improve our services and would be grateful if you could help by telling us where we are satisfactory and where we could improve. All your answers will be treated in confidence but will be considered.

Thank you for taking the time to complete this survey.

Please ring the number that indicates how you feel about each aspect below.
Ring 1 if you felt it was very poor, 2 = poor, 3 = acceptable, 4 = good, 5 = very good/excellent. Please add comments or write overleaf if you wish to say more.

Item			Score		
1. Decoration and appearance of salon	1	2	3	4	5
2. Comfort and cleanliness	1	2	3	4	5
3. Music and lighting	1	2	3	4	5
4. Refreshments and reading	1	2	3	4	5
5. Efficiency of service	1	2	3	4	5
6. Friendliness of staff	1	2	3	4	5
7. Quality of hairdressing service	1	2	3	4	5
8. Were the staff informative about our services and products?	1	2	3	4	5

Will you visit the salon again?   Yes   No   If no, why not?

What things do you like about this salon? ....
....

What do you think could be improved? ....
....

What did you have done today? ....

Which members of staff served you today?..
....

Were you offered any home care products today? ....

Were you told about any promotions we have on offer? ....
....

Thank you for taking the time to complete this survey.

Figure 4.1 Sample client satisfaction survey

Another way of measuring the quality of service is by using a mystery shopper. Someone unknown to the staff will come in and experience the whole customer service package and report back to you. You need to give the mystery shopper a brief and get them to carry out the visits over variety of days and times. Any feedback, positive or negative, needs to be discussed at team meetings and communicated in a constructive way.

Remember that you are continuously trying to improve your quality of service so that you remain the best and can develop the business further.

Improving customer service

The following survey will help you to determine more information about you and your client. It will help to evaluate your personal effectiveness and to identify your training needs. The client data will help you to define your target market and also to expand that market by developing your niche and advertising it. The marketing mix is being able to match these characteristics to products and services, price, place, promotion and combining elements of the mix.

CLIENT SURVEY ASSIGNMENT

Develop and improve personal effectiveness within the job role.

This task requires you to design and conduct a client survey. With your employer's permission, this can be conducted in your salon or, if preferred, in the college/training centre salon. In this case you will need to liaise with reception.

A. Choose the following objectives for your survey:
  ▶ type of client – age/gender
  ▶ number and type of chemical work performed
  ▶ number of new and regular clients
  ▶ number of conversions, e.g. cut and blow dry clients becoming colour, cut & blow dry clients
  ▶ average spend
  ▶ client satisfaction.

B. Design your data collection form to obtain the information. This is likely to be in the form of a client questionnaire. These questionnaires should be completed during interviews with clients, and will either be observed by your assessor or you will need to supply signed witness testimonies from your workplace.

C. Write up a plan of how you intend to implement your survey. Including the following:
  ▶ time scale
  ▶ quantity of clients
  ▶ responsibilities of each salon team member
  ▶ collection arrangements.

D. Conduct your survey in accordance with your plan.

E. Design a spreadsheet to analyse your results.

F. Present your results in a written report, which should incorporate a breakdown of the data that should be described using:
  ▶ simple percentages
  ▶ simple fractions
  ▶ simple decimal fractions
  ▶ simple ratios
  ▶ negative numbers where applicable.

G. You should also include two labelled bar charts and two simple line graphs (to scale) when presenting your results.

H. If your survey was conducted in your salon, present your findings to your manager and the salon team. Discuss any problems identified and ways in which these can be rectified.

This assignment is intended to be positive. Encourage the team to be proactive in what the salon philosophy and business objectives are set to achieve. It is good to remind the team why you are in business, and of the mission statement to keep staff focused in retaining the salon identity.

Reporting changes within client services

Monitor and evaluate the changes in customer services by identifying the impact of quality improvements by looking at sales, percentage customer services, e.g. cut, colour, perm, etc. Run questionnaires at intervals so that you can compare like with like. This way you can evaluate how you are performing and set performance targets for you and your staff. Everyone will benefit as a result.

Review Questions

1   What types of questions are needed in a customer satisfaction survey?

2   Why should the questionnaire be quick for the client to complete?

3   What do we mean by a mystery shopper?

4   What do we mean by a quality service?

5   Why should we monitor performance?

6   State your salon mission statement.

5 UNIT G11 CONTRIBUTE TO THE FINANCIAL EFFECTIVENESS OF THE BUSINESS

1 Contribute to the effectiveness of the business by using and monitoring resources

2 Meet productivity and development targets

CHAPTER CONTENTS

- Continuous Improvement Cycle
- Planning for Improvement
- Your Role In Contributing to the Development of Teams and Individuals
- Identifying Development Needs for Individuals and Teams in Line with Salon Needs
- Producing a Skills/Development Matrix
- Encouraging Individuals and Teams to Identify their Development Needs
- How People Learn

- How to Manage Appropriate Equality of Access to Development
- Performance Review – Good Practice
- Individual Development Plans
- Assessing Development
- Summary
- Further Development Activities
- Review Questions
- Additional information

Introduction

Effective communication is the cornerstone of managing people's performance. People at work are more effective when they have a clear understanding of what is expected of them and they are provided with the appropriate support and encouragement to achieve this. Effective performance management clearly links the activities of the entire salon's staff with the overall aspirations of the salon.

Aspirations of the salon may include becoming recognised as a fashion leader, consolidating the business, increasing levels of turnover, raising profit margins, growing the salon, changing the salon image with clients and/or other hairdressers, and developing into additional or differing aspects of the hairdressing industry.

Staff are the single most important asset of a hairdressing salon. In order for the salon to achieve its plans it is essential that its entire team are aware (at a level appropriate to their needs) of these plans and are all working in the same direction and supporting each other. A single person not working in the appropriate direction can cause the salon to take longer than necessary to achieve its plans or not to achieve its plans at all.

This section will provide you with guidance in the practice of performance management. You will be introduced to how you can influence people's performance at work through effective management and how this, when linked to the salon's plans, will support the salon aims to be successful and achieve its objectives.

You will be provided with guidance on how to:

- draw up salon, team and individual targets from the salon's plans
- undertake performance reviews with individual members of your team
- support and encourage team and individual development
- develop and nurture a culture of continuous professional development.

You will find this section will be most supportive if it is studied in its entirety, as many of the described activities link and can occur concurrently within management interventions.

Continuous improvement cycle

Improvement in the performance of anything can be something that occurs by chance or it can be guided and informed. Leaving improvement to chance may mean that it does not consistently occur, fails to occur within those areas where it is essential, or goes unnoticed and therefore not capitalised upon when it does occur. The continuous improvement cycle is a framework for development to ensure that appropriate actions occur. The cycle has three essential stages, and these are:

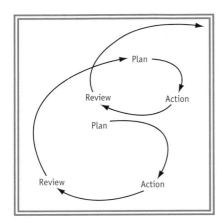

- plan
- action
- review.

Figure 5.1 The continuous improvement cycle

Planning for improvement

You should plan for change and improvement. Your planning will need to state clearly what it hopes to achieve by the change or improvement, how the achievement of this will be measured and what actions are necessary. What is hoped to be achieved is often referred to as the aim. To be able to recognise whether the aim has been achieved you should set targets. These targets will be those things that you would expect to see when the aim has been achieved. Achieving the targets will indicate that the aim has been achieved. Targets will be more effective if they are clearly SMARTER.

S – Specific – stated – stretching
M – Measurable
A – Achievable
R – Relevant
T – Time bound
E – Evaluated
R – Resourced

The actions that are considered necessary to achieve the aims require planning in a sequential manner. This becomes the operational plan:

Remember: Plans should be responsive to the need and you should be prepared to review your plans at appropriate intervals.

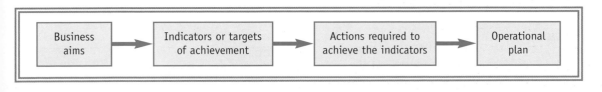

| Business aims | → | Indicators or targets of achievement | → | Actions required to achieve the indicators | → | Operational plan |

Figure 5.2 Planning for change and improvement

Here is an example of an aim linked to SMARTER targets. The salon's aim is to:

- increase the salon turnover by 20% by increasing sales and client services.

The targets or indicators may be identified as:

- increasing client services by 10% and retail by 10% within three months
- increasing client services by 20% and retail by 20% within six months
- increasing the salon turnover by 20% within the next six months
- to be confirmed from an evaluation of the salon's weekly takings
- staff meeting time will be allocated to agree how to increase sales and services and the weekly budget for retail stock will be increased by 5% as improvement is confirmed.

These targets are:

- Specific – they relate to a defined event or occurrence
- Measurable – the number of occurrences is quantifiable
- Achievable – this may be considered realistic for the stylist
- Relevant – the targets would indicate a level of salon recognition
- Time bound – a time frame is stated
- Evaluated – via an audit of weekly takings
- Resourced – time for staff development and increased spend on stock for resale.

The operational plan guides the actions necessary to achieve these planned targets. Effective communication and adequate resources are essential to ensure that the actions take place. You should ensure that those with responsibilities for actions are aware of these requirements sufficiently in advance for any preparations to be made. Adequate resources of time, staffing and materials must be made available at the appropriate times. Resources usually have a financial implication. You may be able to allocate these resources or you may have to discuss their allocation with your line manager.

Evaluation will confirm if and when the aim has been achieved. Evaluation is simply the process of gathering relevant information together to judge to what extent a target has been met. Through evaluation lessons may be learned, which may include:

- confirmation, or not, that the aim has been achieved (measurement against the SMARTER targets previously set)
- what, if any, further actions are required in order to achieve the aim
- potential improvements to make future actions more effective
- what has changed or been gained as a result of the actions.

On-going monitoring provides the information that enables evaluation to take place.

Within your hairdressing salon the continuous improvement cycle may be used as part of the process of developing the salon at all levels:

- supporting the salon development as a whole by increasing the salon turnover
- supporting the teams' development by taking responsibility as a team member
- supporting an individual's training or development by sharing good practice and development.

Remember: Being too busy to evaluate actions can often result in wasted effort or unnecessary or inappropriate actions being taken.

The process of continuous improvement creates a sound culture for the consistent, cohesive development of all people and activity within the hairdressing business.

Your role in contributing to the development of teams and individuals

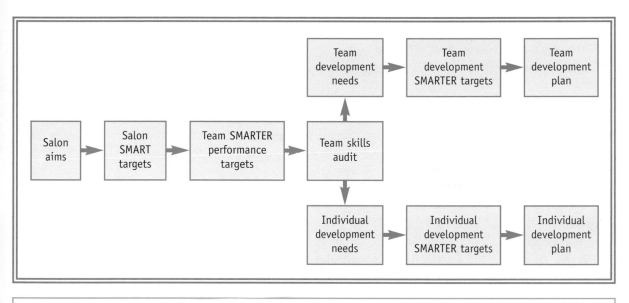

Figure 5.3 Team development chart

Identifying development needs for individuals and teams in line with salon needs

As a person with responsibility for the line management of teams and individuals your role will include developing the skills, knowledge and attitudes in line with the salon needs. In planning to contribute to the development of a team and its individual members you will need to have a clear understanding of the team's objectives. The objectives will have cascaded down from the business plan and will be the performance targets and indicators for the team that support the achievement of the salon's overall aims. Objectives that are SMARTER will be clearly defined and you will be able to recognise and confirm when they are achieved.

The development needs are those actions that are required to develop the team from their current position on skills, knowledge and attitudes, to a position that meets the SMARTER objectives. Having identified the development needs you may then determine if they are whole team developments or the development of differing team members to support the whole team achievement. Within hairdressing salons individuals often have differing roles and responsibilities within the team, as opposed to all team members having identical roles.

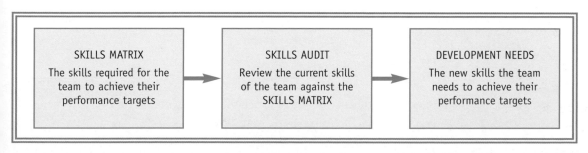

Figure 5.4 Identifying development needs

Producing a skills/development matrix

A useful starting point is to produce a matrix of the skills, knowledge and attitudes that are needed within a team and its individuals in order that the team's objectives can be achieved. An audit of individuals and the team against these will help you objectively identify development areas. The audit should be approached as the opportunity to support individuals and teams, not as a judgemental or critical process. Within a salon team there needs to be a balance of skills, and not all staff need specialist skills, for example hair extensions, therefore within the team matrix only a limited number of the team may be targeted with that development. However, the salon will wish to ensure it has sufficient team members able to provide hair extensions to satisfy the clients' needs and to ensure continuity should a member of staff leave employment in the salon. Skills for effective communication will be required of all team members; therefore it would appear on each person's skills matrix.

To gain acceptance of this process you should involve team members in the identification of the skills, knowledge and attitudes required of their team in order to meet its plans. The criteria that are identified within the matrix will be best stated as measurable outcomes or behaviour rather than vague statements open to wide interpretation.

For example, if your and your team performance targets are to introduce Indian Head Massage as a service to clients within the next three months, and you expect this to represent 10% of the team's income, you will first need to understand what skills knowledge and approaches are required to offer this service – the **skills matrix**. You and your team undertake an audit of what skills and knowledge your team currently has – i.e. an **audit**. For those that are missing you will plan to develop in the most effective manner possible – the **development plan**. Some development may be common for all of the team, possibly background knowledge of the massage process, its features and benefits – **team development needs**. Some development may be required only by a single person, say the actual massage skills – **individual development needs**. To increase your turnover by 10% where your current average client spend per visit is £75, your clients would need to increase their spend £7.50. For every 100 clients visiting the salon each week, this additional spend would generate an additional income of £750 per week.

Encouraging individuals and teams to identify their development needs

While you will undertake a review of your team and individuals against the criteria of the matrix, you should also provide an opportunity for the team to undertake a review against the matrix both collectively and individually. Including team members will make the process more effective as:

- there will be a greater resource of ideas
- people will feel less threatened when being reviewed against a matrix to which they have contributed
- people will understand why they are being reviewed
- people will more readily accept the findings of the review.

When the overall development needs for the team and its individuals have been determined you will be able to plan how these will be met. You should consider:

- developments that are for the team and those for individuals
- links to the overall plan for the salon
- priority areas for development
- sequence of development (some development may need to occur before subsequent activity can occur)
- what it is hoped will be achieved as a result of the development (SMARTER target) and how, when and by whom this will be reviewed
- how the development will occur

- the cost implications
- the person to be responsible to initiate the development activity.

The team must be proactive in successfully meeting targets set, therefore it is important they consider how their effective development will impact on this success.

Having identified development needs and their planned impact upon the salon you will be aware of the impact on the salon of not implementing them. This will help you in determining the level of priority that a development activity should be given.

How people learn

People develop skills, knowledge and attitudes in many different ways. In planning for development you will need to consider the range of development opportunities and determine the most appropriate. Considering the impact of previous development activity can often provide guidance when considering alternatives. Influencing factors include:

- preferred learning styles
- the development requirement
- costs and budget available
- time available, lost income
- resources available within the salon
- resources available outside of the salon.

How different people develop

Development can occur as the result of a wide range of actions. It does not always require an external training course to achieve an identified required outcome. In some cases simply ensuring that an individual is fully aware of your expectations can be sufficient for development to occur. Consider the range of development opportunities, including:

- discussion and attending meetings
- reading books and magazines, watching training videos
- watching others at work – shadowing
- undertaking new tasks – experiential learning
- working with study guides – paper or computer-based
- visiting exhibitions and hairdressing shows
- training sessions within the salon, provided by salon staff or external trainers
- training sessions located externally at training centres, colleges and academies.

Individuals and teams often have preferred learning styles – the way they learn most effectively. In most cases people learn most effectively when they are actively involved in the process. Passive learning often results in short-term development. When planning development activities you should consult with those who will be undertaking them to determine their preferences and previous experiences. Use your findings to guide your decision. Previous adverse experiences can place barriers to development. Previous successful experiences may indicate that person's preferred learning style. You may also wish to consult with others who may have undertaken similar development to gain their opinions of experiences.

Some forms of development have obvious cost implications, for example course fees. For others the cost may be embedded in the time taken away from work with paying clients. You may reduce the cost implication by utilising times when the salon is less busy. Building on the skills that already exist within the salon is often effective not only in cost saving but also in building an individual's self-esteem. Some manufacturing and wholesaling companies provide training in their product usage free of charge to salons. Talk to sales representatives visiting your salon to find out more about this opportunity. When a number of people require the same development it may be more cost effective to arrange for a trainer to visit the salon in preference to everyone travelling to a training centre. When considering this option ensure, if appropriate, that there will be adequate equipment or material available for all to use.

With a wide range of options you may wish to obtain guidance in selecting the most appropriate. Training consultants can provide this advice. Contact a range of training organisations and obtain their prospectus so that you are aware of what is available. Your local Learning and Skills Council, Business Link and HABIA (Hairdressing and Beauty Industry Authority) can provide guidance about the range of training and development opportunities available. When you are fully aware of the options available and the features of each, you will be able to judge what is the most appropriate. Discuss your plans with your line manager before introducing them to your team or individuals.

You should discuss planned group development activities with the group, as a whole. An individual's development will usually be discussed within their confidential review or an interim meeting.

How to manage appropriate equality of access to development

By linking your people development activity to the needs of the salon you will be providing fair access to development. The determination of the need and subsequent development activity is based upon a clear criteria of the needs of the salon. Communicate this to all of your staff so that they are aware of why certain interventions are given priority over others. You should avoid being pressured into providing training that is not in line with the salon needs. If you are in doubt, seek advice from your line manager and consider its priority against other identified staff development needs.

Performance review – good practice

Performance review can occur at all levels within the hairdressing salon – at whole salon level, team level, and individual level. This section will focus on the team and individual.

At individual level, you will typically undertake this review as a confidential, one-to-one meeting between yourself and the individual. This process is sometimes known as appraisal. The purpose of this meeting is twofold – to reflect on the past and to plan for the future. You should steer the meeting to reflect on previous work actions and achievements, identify and recognise good practice as well as focusing on less successful activity. This reflection will support the person

Remember: A performance review meeting is not normally an appropriate time to undertake disciplinary issues or to issue reprimands. These should be dealt with separately.

being reviewed to build on existing good practice and to learn from mistakes. When reflecting on previous less successful activity, you should take into account the influence of any external factors there may have been, such as periods of heavy workload due to a colleague's absence, lack of suitable consumable stock or equipment, or high levels of local unemployment.

Planning for the future will be guided by the priorities for the salon that have been identified through the business planning process. An individual's planning focuses on their role in supporting the salon in its priorities and will involve both of you agreeing targets of achievement for the future. These targets may relate to:

- changes in working practices, attitudes or behaviour
- volume of clients that the individual will work with
- ratio of conversions of client services from basic hairstyling to chemical processes
- developing specific hairdressing skills.

These are just a few examples. Targets should, wherever possible, be SMARTER.

As well as identifying targets your planning will consider changes in the individual's job role, identified development needs and how they may be met.

The performance review meeting should be a two-way dialogue, providing ample opportunity and encouragement for the person being reviewed to contribute. In order to support the individual in their preparation for the review, provide the individual with a pre-meeting self review document that can guide them in preparing their thoughts. If you do not work closely with the person you are reviewing it may be appropriate to obtain information about their performance from their supervisor and from any available management information and customer feedback.

> *Remember: For a performance review to be successful you should obtain sufficient information about the individual, their role, performance and salon plans prior to the meeting.*

Give sufficient advance notice; agree a mutually convenient time for the meeting and set aside sufficient uninterrupted meeting time. It is often best if the meeting takes place in a location that is neutral to both you, the reviewer, and the person being reviewed. If this is not possible the meeting should take place in a setting that is not intimidating. Avoid large barriers (for example, tables) between participants, avoid seating at differing heights. Ensure both people are seated comfortably.

> *Remember: A performance review is a positive, supportive process designed to support and encourage the individual in their performance at work.*

The meeting will be successful if agreement is reached regarding:

- previous performance levels
- targets for future performance/achievement
- changing or developing work roles (if appropriate)
- identified training and development actions.

You may decide to record your agreements. This may appear to make the meeting more formal but it will provide a record to which you may both refer. If a written record is made, it is usual for both people to sign and date it and for a copy to be retained by both. Ensure that an individual's training and development plans are agreed and updated (more guidance is provided later in this section) and that relevant information is passed to those who will be responsible for facilitating these actions.

Your salon may have pre-set forms for recording the agreements of the review. Ensure that these are completed legibly, appropriately, within the required timescale and passed only to those authorised. The discussions within the review meeting should be considered confidential and should not be discussed with any unauthorised person. The information that you hold about individuals of your team are subject to the conditions of the Data Protection Act (see Chapter 3).

Individual review meetings may occur as frequently as required, but at least once a year. Often a formal review occurs once a year with interim less formal reviews between. It is important for confidence in the process to be developed. Any identified and agreed actions should be implemented within the agreed timescale. If plans have to be changed, you should inform the individuals affected of the reasons and any planned alternatives.

> *Remember: Be honest with your feedback within review, as being less than honest can cause problems at a later stage when remedial actions are required.*

At team level the review may take the form of a guided team meeting where you encourage the team to reflect on their previous actions and achievement. Within a team review meeting, as with any group meeting, you should ensure that all those you wish to attend are given sufficient notice and are aware of its level of priority above other work-related activity. Everyone attending the meeting should be aware of what the meeting is trying to achieve, and should be encouraged to contribute. People may be encouraged to participate if:

- they feel that their point of view will be valued

- they are not afraid of being ridiculed for their opinion

- adequate time is given for all to contribute

- negative constructive opinions are received without apportioning blame.

> **Remember:** *An individual's participation within team evaluations can develop team spirit and feelings of inclusion and responsibility.*

Avoid unhelpful interruption or digressions that can consume valuable meeting time. You should allocate time for discussion and suggest that discussions that are not relevant are facilitated at another time. Ensure that the meetings end at the agreed time so that all who wish to contribute are able to and others can respond. Before concluding the meeting summarise the findings, confirm any agreements and planned actions, and state who will be responsible for their implementation.

A written record of the meeting or of the agreements and actions to be taken can be a useful tool when reviewing progress and keeping planned actions on track.

Individual development plans

Plans for an individual's development provide a recorded schedule of activities clearly stated for the benefit of the individual and the person with responsibility for implementation. In some cases the individual may hold the responsibility for implementing the identified development activities. The plan also provides an arbitrating document when reviewing activities and the achievement of targets.

You will update the plan following a formal or interim review. It should also be updated at any time when a training or development activity is identified or evaluated.

Typically, the detail included within the development plan is:

- the proposed development activity

- the required outcome of the activity (SMARTER target)

- the person responsible for implementation

- how, when and by whom the outcome will be evaluated

- record of the evaluation.

An individual's development plan usually feeds into their overall career plan. You should encourage all staff to have a career plan. This is their long-term development plan and encourages individuals to be strategic in their development. Plans of this nature nurture a culture of development, encouraging individuals to personally review their actions and development needs.

INDIVIDUAL DEVELOPMENT PLAN

Name *Alison Brown*   Job role *Hair stylist*

Development activity
When time permits work with Joanna on hair extensions. Use your Monday training time to work on the training head using hair extensions. A practice kit and fibre will be provided. Salon manager to arrange with Joanna and ensure materials are available.

Outcomes
You are able to provide hair extensions to your own clients without the help of Joanna. By February your salon taking increase by an average of 10% due to hair extension work. To be reviewed at the March performance review.

Evaluation
To date weekly takings have increased by 6%. Some issues regarding availability of suitable fibre. The salon will increase the stock of fibre. To be reviewed at the June review

Signed *Alison Brown*   Date *10 March 2003*
Signed *Mary Higgs*   Date *10 March 2003*

Figure 5.5 A sample individual development plan

Assessing development

A prerequisite for effective evaluation is the agreement of targets for outcomes that are SMARTER. Evaluation is not focused if the required outcome of an activity (what is wished to be achieved as the result) is not determined before the activity is undertaken. Remember the importance of utilising resources effectively and efficiently. So much profit is lost through wastage and lack of control. It is not efficient to increase the salon turnover by 20% if it has cost almost that in training, time, effort and resources.

Before any individual or team undertakes a development activity you should ensure that participants have a clear understanding of why they are undertaking the task, what is hoped to be achieved as a result and how this will be implemented in their work. Participants will be better able to achieve the desired result if they are quite clear about what it is. How this communication occurs is determined by you, the organisation and the individual situation. Often this discussion will occur within an individual's review or, for a team, within a staff team meeting. For development identified outside of the review meeting, additional discussion may take place.

Following the development activity you will assess, with the individual, whether they have gained the necessary skills, knowledge or understanding to be able to implement this development in their normal working activity. The assessment may take the form of your observation of a task in a training situation, the results from a brief written test, a discussion or a combination of these. The selected assessment method will depend upon the nature of the change. You should feed back the findings of the assessment to the individual or team to ensure full understanding and, if necessary, identify any further action necessary to achieve the overall desired result.

The feedback sandwich

For feedback to have a positive effect follow these steps:

- Identify achievements and quantify good practice.
- Identify areas for further development (no blame), improvements, or change. Include SMARTER targets. Give clear guidance of exactly what is required.
- Identify positive future steps and confirm next actions.
- Summarise.
- Gain agreement.

Within an agreed timescale you will undertake an evaluation of the impact of the development on work. This evaluation may take the form of observation of working practices, reviewing performance through management information data or client feedback. The impacts of development should be shared with the individual and they should be encouraged to view the impact of their actions on their team's performance and that of the salon as a whole. This awareness will build an individual's self-esteem and develop their awareness of the importance of their actions to the success of the team and the salon.

It is very likely that your line manager will wish to be kept informed of the impact that development has upon the performance of individuals, teams and the salon. Recording the findings of evaluation on the individual's development plan will help to inform future decisions about development activities, as well as informing future performance reviews.

Summary

This section has provided you with an overview of performance management and your role in contributing to the effectiveness of the business in line with the salon's plans. You will be aware that as an employee/manager you have a responsibility to support your team in working effectively. This includes providing guidance in good working practices, honestly providing regular and timely feedback about performance and providing support for the development skills, knowledge and attitudes in line with the salon's plans.

Further development activities

You will wish to develop and practise the skills of people management and development. You may require the co-operation and support of your line manager to provide the opportunity to undertake these tasks. Initially you may find it supportive to observe or sit in on an individual's review. When you attend team meetings observe how they are managed and reflect on what you see. Model your own practice on good practice that you see, and learn from those practices that appear less effective.

When you initially undertake these activities you may find referring to a task analysis or a list of essential points helpful to ensure effective performance. If you do not have the appropriate answers be honest about this and undertake to find out and report back. Once you are competent you may present evidence of your activity for assessment and recognition. Some of your activities may have been confidential. Confidentiality must be maintained or permission obtained from those concerned before this is breached. You should discuss your proposal, and plan how you will undertake the presentation of evidence with your own assessor.

Review Questions

1 What are SMARTER targets?

2 What is meant by the term 'the continuous improvement cycle'?

3 What is evaluation?

4 Why use a team skills matrix and what will it provide?

5 State two benefits to be gained from involving others in the identification of a team skills matrix.

6 State one way that individuals can be encouraged to accept the findings of a review against a skills matrix.

7 State four items to be considered when planning to meet individual and team development needs.

8 State six different development techniques.

9 Who can you approach for guidance and advice in training?

10 What four aspects should be agreed within a successful performance review?

Additional information

Useful websites

Website Addresses	Content
www.habia.org.uk	Hairdressing and Beauty Industry Authority. Downloads available including references to other websites
www.bbc-safety.co.uk	Free advice on diseases in hairdressing
www.lookfantastic.com	Professional hairdressing products and advice
www.laurandp.co.uk	Educational publications for development of professional hairdressing
www.dti.gov.uk	Department of Trade and Industry
www.cipd.org.uk	Chartered Institute of Personnel and Development

Magazines and journals

- *Hairdressers Journal*
- *Creative Head*
- *Estetica/Cutting Edge*
- *Black Beauty and Hair*

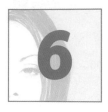

6 UNIT H19 PROVIDE SHAVING SERVICES

1 Maintain effective and safe methods of working when shaving

2 Prepare the hair and skin for shaving

3 Shave hair

CHAPTER CONTENTS

- Safe Working Practices
- Client Care
- Client Consultation
- Facial Features
- Assessing the Hair
- Preparing for the Shave
- Preparing Razors for Use
- Facial Shaving
- Outline Shaving
- Review Questions
- Additional Information
- Activity

Introduction

The traditional art of the barber includes that of shaving and face massage. Shaving in barber shops used to be extremely popular. In fact most traditional barbering has been around for over 2000 years. Evidence of shaving the beard may be found in the earliest civilisations. Men used to visit the barber daily for a regular shave. Nowadays, this may appear to be a skill that is no longer relevant. The introduction of the safety razor and electric razor has caused a decline of the professional shaving service in barber salons over the last few decades. However, these skills are undergoing a renaissance. Wet shaving is a skill that is still in demand within certain communities and geographic areas. The purpose of shaving is to remove visible hair, leaving the skin smooth to touch. Shaving is used to remove unwanted hair mainly from the face and neck on men. Fashions in facial hair have required the skill of outline shaving as part of the shaping process. The skills of shaving may also be applied to the art of shaved

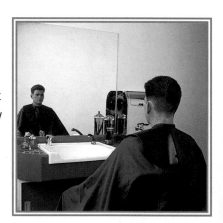

Figure 6.1 Client awaiting showing services

partings, used with afro-Caribbean hair, to define a parting in short hair. Shaved outlines, used to define the hairline in sculptured designs, around the ears and in the nape as well as shapes shaved in the hairlines, all require control in the execution to produce the finish achieved. Facial massage is usually coupled with the shaving process. It is a traditional barbering skill that may be used to relax your client and give him a feeling of well-being.

Men today seem to like the convenience of being able to shave in the comfort of their own home as so many lead a busy lifestyle and time is of the essence. Some men also like to be pampered and, in particular, those who have important meetings or special occasions to go to really do value the personal touch of a professional shaving service.

If this service is provided well in a professional relaxing environment you will find that the client will want to book again.

What better way to start the day than by giving a complete service that leaves the client looking and feeling good? When complemented by a facial massage and the correct advice on skincare products, this gives him the confidence to carry out his day-to-day duties. The emphasis has to be on the 'the professional service' when shaving is done well. That is why we need to make sure that the client does have a really good experience and feels confident in your capable hands. So where do we start?

Safe working practices

The number one priority is health and safety:

- Wear suitable, clean and safe clothing. Any open cuts or sores on your hands must be covered with a waterproof dressing.

- Prevent cross infection by using clean tools and equipment, disposable razors, sterilising liquids, tissue paper, clean towels, brushes, disposable sponges, etc. Wear protective tight-fitting fine rubber gloves in order to use the razor and to tension the skin effectively.

- Check for symptoms of non-infectious conditions including psoriasis and eczema as you will need to take care not to cut the client in these areas where the skin's surface will be irregular.

- Check for symptoms of infectious conditions including tinea capitis, folliculitus and impetigo. Clients with these conditions should be referred to a general practitioner and should not be treated in the salon. See Chapter 3 for further information.

- Open razors are very sharp and must always be treated with care and respect. Reduce risk by keeping the handle closed to cover the blade when not in use, when passing it, and when carrying it. If passing the razor to a colleague, do so with the tang facing away from you, being careful to prevent it opening. Never place a razor in your pocket. Always keep razors away from children.

- Always check the temperature of the hot steam towel before wrapping it on the client to ensure it isn't too hot, as each client's tolerance of heat on the skin differs. Ensure that steam towels are not too wet as this may scald.

- To prevent cross infection use separate soap blocks or powdered/liquid/gel soaps. Ensure lather brushes are clean and sterile for each client.

- A new sponge must be used for each client.

- The skin must always be stretched taut before carrying out the stroke with the razor to prevent cutting the client.

- Do not shave the hair too close to the skin as it could cause irritation and ingrown hairs (particularly with curly hair).

- Finish the shave by using an antiseptic, moisturiser or talcum powder to smooth the skin. An aftershave lotion or balm may be used as an astringent to close the pores of the skin.

- A different fixed blade razor should be used for each client. Fixed blade razors must always be sterilised before use.

- Sterilise equipment after use including scissors, clippers, combs, razors, etc, using radiation, autoclaves and chemical methods. Ensure all tools are clean before use. Further information in Chapter 1. Always sterilise razors after stropping.

- Dispose of sharps correctly in a sharps disposable box, following your salon policy.

- Soiled disposable materials should be placed in a sealed plastic bag for removal following your salon policy.

- Check with your local council whether you are allowed to use a fixed blade razor as they are prohibited in many areas. Detachable blades are better as they are disposable. If using detachable blades, a new blade must be fitted for each client.

- High standards of hygienic practice are paramount to the success of shaving services in your salon. Ensure your client understands these precautions are always carried out.

- Ensure you know how to access the first-aid kit and keep yourself up to date with the salon's first-aid procedures.

First-aid materials should always be available. For nicks and cuts use styptic liquid or powder. You can use a styptic pen but you must renew it for each client.

- Tidy up after yourself.

Legal responsibilities

As barbers/hairdressers you have a legal responsibility to your clients and employers with regard to your own responsibilities for health, safety, security, promotion and sales of foods and services, and handling client information. Information about these Acts is provided in Chapters 1 and 2.

Types of sterilisation

Sterilisation is the process of destroying all organisms whether harmful or not. There are several methods of sterilisation: moist heat, dry heat, radiation, vapours and disinfectants. For more information see Unit G1.

Client care

Client safety and comfort should be assured. With any service you should provide the correct protection. This should be done by gowning the client to stop hairs and products falling on their clothes, reducing any discomfort and risk of damaging their personal belongings. The client should feel comfortable at all times to ensure they experience a good professional service, e.g. sitting the client at the right height so that you can carry out the service safely and effectively.

Client consultation

Your client should be consulted and agreement reached on the service, taking into consideration their personal views and eliciting the correct information so that the client is satisfied with the end result. You can do this by keeping updated records and referring to them as and when needed, and advising the client on what is important and what will suit them. Use visual aids, e.g. magazines, photographs of current and emerging trends, with the correct aftercare advice. Suggest other services that might be of interest to them.

You must check their facial skin and hair types so that you can use products that suit the client and the purpose. Some clients are particularly sensitive to products when shaving so using the right soap for lathering and the correct moisturisers are important as you do not want your client leaving the salon with a reaction causing the skin to become red or blemished. Checking for contra indications is important, therefore the consultation needs to be thorough. A consultation sheet on which you record the information is useful, and ensures that you have not missed anything out.

Your perception of the end result may differ to that of your client so it is always best to summarise and agree exactly what you are going to do. This reassures your client and makes them feel in safe hands. Ask your client the following and decide:

1. What does the client want?
2. What type of shaving service would he like?
3. Does he have any condition that may prevent you from shaving and if so what will you recommend?
4. Does he want a close shave?
5. Does he have a moustache? Does he want to keep it? If yes, what shape, etc?
6. Does he have a beard? Does he want to keep it? If yes, what shape, etc?
7. Does he have sideburns? Does he want to keep them? If yes, what shape, etc?
8. What skin type does he have?
9. What type of hair does he have?
10. How often does he shave? How does he usually shave?

11 Does he have any problems when shaving? If so, what problems?

12 Does he have any scars, broken skin or abnormalities in the area that may affect the end result?

13 What types of hair growth patterns does he have?

14 Look for areas that are dense or fine, etc.

15 What hair texture does he have – curly, strong, coarse, etc?

16 What are his facial features and the balance between these?

17 What shapes would he like to compliment his looks?

More aspects of client consultation are reviewed in Chapter 3.

Facial features

The distribution of hair and the shape you create is important, as this can really affect the overall look and balance. It is extremely personal and once you have removed the hair it could take some time to grow back. Time given to looking at these features is time well spent, as each person is totally different, with varying combinations of:

- mouth shape
- width of the top lip
- nose shape
- amount of space between the nose and the lip
- shape of the jaw and chin
- breadth and the depth of the jaw and chin
- jaw line
- chin and the amount of flesh around this area
- distinguishing marks, e.g. moles, birthmarks etc.

Assessing the hair

Density of the hair

The amount of hair will affect the shave. If the hair is very dense (large amount of hairs that grow in a given area of the skin) you may need to shave a 'second time over' shave. Men with very dense hair may need to shave twice a day. The term 'blue beard' is given to men who have very dense beards as the skin still appears to have a tinge of blue after shaving.

Younger men often have sparse facial hair growth, which becomes denser as they become older.

Texture of the hair

Hair can be fine, medium or coarse. Coarse hair can be very difficult to shave. You will have to lather the area and massage it more to help soften the hair prior to shaving.

Fine hair is easier to razor as it doesn't cause too much resistance. Often as men get older the hair tends to become coarser. Your choice of razor may be influenced by the hair's texture.

Preparing for the shave

Once you have decided what you are going to do and how you are going to do it, you will need to make sure you are fully prepared. Prepare well as there is nothing worse than leaving your client once you have started because you have forgotten something. Not only does it waste time, it looks unprofessional.

Ensure you have prepared the following:

1. Hot and cool towels prepared or pre-packed.

2. A roll of tissue paper.

3. First-aid materials, styptic liquid or powder or pencil (remember a new one for each client).

4. Tight-fitting protective gloves.

5. Products to carry out the shave – soaps, foam, gel, lubricating oil, aftershaves, lotions, balms, moisturisers and talcum powder.

6. Tools depending on the type of shave to be given. Open razors must be sharpened or set, or a detachable disposable blade, fixed razors that are hollow ground or solid ground, which must be sterilised prior to each client.

7. Hydraulic adjustable chair.

8. A hone and/or strop if you intend to use a fixed razor.

9. Lather brush, mug or bowl if using soaps (remember, you must thoroughly clean the brush in disinfectant and sterilise between clients). You may have the client's own personal shaving brush, bowl and mug. Solid shaving soap blocks must only be used with one client. Powdered soap, soap shavings or gels may be used as only a specific amount is dispensed and any residual should be disposed of.

10. Clean gowns, etc.

Types of Razors

Open razors are also known as cut-throat razors and have a hinged handle that closes to protect the blade when not in use. These are usually used in barbering and can have either a fixed blade or detachable blade.

Fixed blade razors must be sharpened or set and can be hollow, half-hollow, or solid ground. Traditional barbers used these for many years. Commercially they are difficult to use as they have to be sterilised before each client's shave and this can be time consuming

Hollow ground razors may be of either English or German origin. They are made of hardened steel and are concave in appearance when viewed end-on. The steel is prepared by a special heat treatment called tempering. This gives the razor the correct degree of hardening to produce a good cutting edge. Hollow ground razors are usually 'hard tempered', which makes them difficult to sharpen (set) but the sharp edge lasts longer.

Hollow ground razors are light in weight, which gives a much nicer feel and tends to be preferred by most barbers for shaving. They are less suitable for cutting hair.

Solid ground or French razors are made of steel. They are soft tempered and are much heavier and more rigid compared to a hollow ground razor. This makes them easier to sharpen but the sharp edge does not last as long. Owing to the greater weight they are more rigid and therefore more suitable for cutting hair than shaving. Some barbers prefer them for use when shaving delicate skin surfaces.

Detachable razors are designed to be very similar to a hollow ground razor but they have disposable blades that are easily replaced. Barbers usually choose this type of razor because they are more hygienic to use than a fixed blade razor.

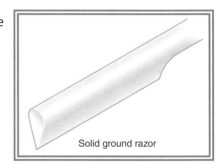
Solid ground razor

Figure 6.2 Solid ground razor

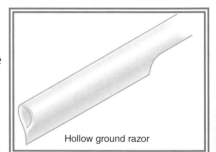
Hollow ground razor

Figure 6.3 Hollow ground razor

Preparing razors for use

Solid ground and hollow ground razors have to be sharpened or set to keep them in good working order. The process of setting a razor is called honing. Honing is a process that requires a great deal of skill to ensure that the edge of the razor is set correctly. The edge of the razor has very fine teeth cut into the blade. These teeth make the blade sharp. The process of honing realigns the old teeth and sets the new teeth into place into the edge of the razor. The simplest way to test the razor is to place it very carefully on a thumb nail. Slowly draw the razor from the heel to the toe of the razor. If there are any snags and the razor doesn't grip and tug smoothly then you will need to sharpen again. Be careful not to damage the razor by over honing. Test the sharpness of the razor frequently.

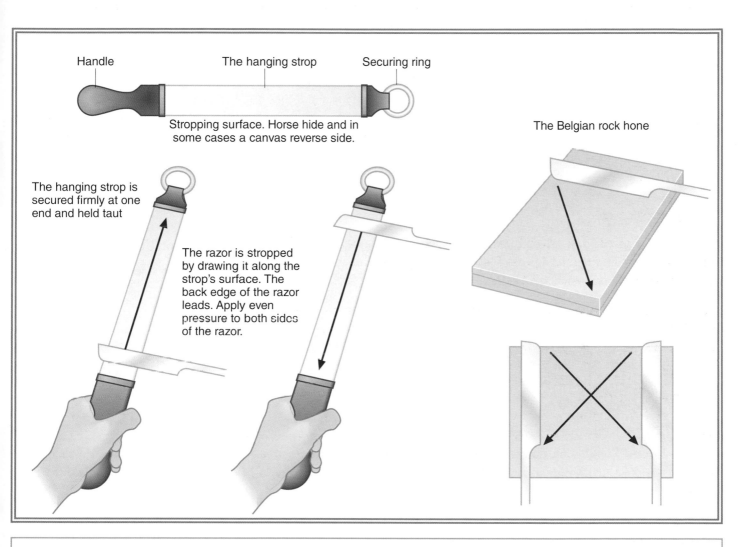

Handle   The hanging strop   Securing ring

Stropping surface. Horse hide and in some cases a canvas reverse side.

The Belgian rock hone

The hanging strop is secured firmly at one end and held taut

The razor is stropped by drawing it along the strop's surface. The back edge of the razor leads. Apply even pressure to both sides of the razor.

Figure 6.4 Stropping

Hones

There are various types of hones available for sharpening razors. These usually consist of a rectangular block of abrasive material that is harder than the razor itself. It is because of this hardness that it has the ability to sharpen.

Natural hones come from naturally occurring rock. These have to be lubricated by water, lather or fine oil before use and have a slow moving, cutting action that produces a fine edge which is long lasting.

Water hones are natural and are from Germany and Belgium.

Synthetic hones are man-made and can be used either wet or dry. The cutting action is much faster than a natural hone. It is particularly important to test the blade regularly as it is very easy to over hone the blade. A carborundum hone is a popular type of synthetic hone.

The method of setting a hollow ground razor

1. Lubricate the hone as recommended by the manufacturer with water, lather or oil.
2. Place the razor flat on the hone. Face the razor edge towards the middle.
3. Slide the blade lightly across the hone with the blade edge leading. Move the blade diagonally from head to toe.
4. Watch the hand and finger position to consistently acquire the correct pressure and angle.
5. Rotate the razor between the thumb and forefinger. Keep the back of the razor on the hone.
6. Continue to rotate until the blade is pointing upwards.
7. Push the razor away from your body upwards until the heel is level with the bottom edge of the hone.
8. Continue rotating the razor as before until the blade is flat, with its edge facing the middle of the hone.
9. Slide the blade diagonally from heel to toe.
10. Repeat these movements several times.
11. Every few strokes ensure you test the blade so as not to overhone the razor.

Stropping fixed blade razors

Stropping a razor does not cut into the steel. Stropping a razor polishes and cleans the edge depending on which side of the strop is used. There are two main types of strops – hanging strops and hand or Hamon strops.

Hanging strops are leather one side (used for polishing) and canvas the other side (used for cleaning). They are mainly used for stropping hollow ground razors. They are designed to hang from a swivel. Hanging strops are popular with barbers.

Hand or Hamon strops are usually made of sprung wood. They are then covered again with balsa wood one side and leather the other side. These are mainly used to strop solid ground razors but tend to be less popular with barbers.

New strops need to be worn in prior to use in order that they are effective. Therefore it is important to follow the manufacturer's instructions. A method frequently used for wearing the strop in is rubbing a pumice stone across the surface to make the surface smooth. Then rub a stiff lather into the canvas surface of the strop and then rub again with the pumice repeatedly. Sweat oil is used on the leather surface. The hand or Hamon strop has its own dressing paste, separate paste for each surface.

Facial shaving

Tools and materials

Tools

Razors

The traditional tool for wet shaving is the open razor, a solid blade of metal pivoting from a handle or shield. The blade of the razor can be made from metal of a variety of degrees of hardness and with one of three cross section shapes (grinds). The grinds are solid or wedge grind, half hollow grind and hollow ground. The solid grind is the earliest shape and produced a rather heavy razor, which could be difficult to manipulate and gave little sensation to the shaver, therefore making it difficult to determine appropriate shaving pressures, etc, to be used. The half hollow grind (French razor) gave a little more sensitivity to the shaver. Made of a soft metal, which made it easier to keep sharp but did not retain the edge, this razor was traditionally used for hair cutting and for shaving fine, delicate beards. The hollow ground (German) razor was most widely used for shaving. Made of very hard steel, which once sharp retained its edge, the finesse of the blade made it responsive to the shaver and easily manipulated across the face.

For commercial shaving these razors are no longer considered hygienically suitable. The difficulty in sterilising the blade's edge made it unsuitable for use when there is a risk of puncturing the skin's surface. They are and may still be used safely when used only on the one individual. For all commercial wet shaving a razor that accepts a disposable blade must be used. There are a number of these commercially available.

They consist of a holder for the blade together with a handle/shield. Some styles accept a double edge blade, snapped in half, and others accept specially prepared blades that are fitted from a dispenser. Disposable razors made in the style of the open razor are also available. Your choice of razor may depend on your salon policy or that which you find the most comfortable to use.

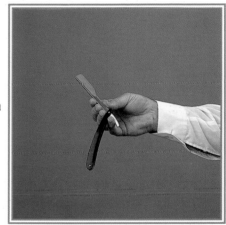

Figure 6.5 A disposable razor in the style of an open raxor

Lather brushes

The best quality lather brushes are said to have bristles of badger hair. However, brushes are available made of both natural and synthetic bristles.

Lather bowls

Clean, sterile bowls are required, one to contain a supply of very hot water in which to warm the lather brush, the second to contain the lather.

Materials

Shaving soap

The solid block of soap must only be used when shaving commercially if it is reserved for use on one client. Powdered shaving soap may be shaken directly onto the bristles of a hot moist lather brush and then applied direct to the face and progressively worked up into a lather. Shaving cream or gel is the more current product used – a small amount is placed into a bowl and then worked into a lather using the lather brush. Aerosol shaving foam is not suitable as working this lather decreases its foam.

Astringent

An astringent is a substance that will close the pores and tighten the skin. Cold water may be used as a mild astringent or aftershave may be used, but take care as the perfume within the lotion may conflict with the cologne use by your client. The stinging effect of aftershave may be reduced by diluting it with water; this is particularly relevant when treating delicate skin. Witch hazel may also be used.

Fine talc

This is used to soothe the skin. The talc should be unperfumed so that it does not clash with your client's cologne.

Coagulant

In case of bleeding a sterile coagulant, powdered Alum BP, or Ferric Chloride is required.

The shaving process

- Preparation of the work area and tools.
- Analysis of the beard area.
- Preparing the face and softening the beard.
- Removing the beard (first time over).
- Re-lathering the beard.
- Removing the beard (second time over).
- Removing remaining lather.
- Closing the pores.
- Cleansing and sterilising tools and materials.

Prepare all tools prior to undertaking the shave on your client. All tools that will make contact with your client's skin must be clean and sterile. An autoclave may be used to sterilise all metal tools, chemical sterilising fluids are used to sterilise those tools which have parts that cannot tolerate high temperatures.

Remember: The autoclave sterilises by steaming items, under pressure, at a temperature of 120°C. Use an autoclave only if you have been trained and following the manufacturer's instructions for safe use.

Check that the hydraulic chair is clean and safe for use. Lock the chair in position at its lowest position, with the back upright and headrest in place. Should your client step onto a hydraulic chair footrest when it is not locked in position, the chair may spin away from your client causing them to fall. This type of chair is in its most stable condition when the hydraulic lift is at its lowest position and is therefore the most suitable position when your client becomes seated. Raise the hydraulic chair to a comfortable working height using the foot or electric pump. Remember to lock the swivel of the chair in place at all times, when adjustment has been completed.

A number of hot steam towels will be required and should be prepared beforehand. Specialist towel steamers are available.

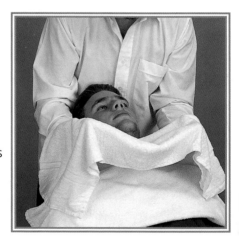

Figure 6.6 The steam towel

A towel is folded in half, lengthwise, and then in half across the length. A small amount of water may be applied to this fold and then the towel is rolled tightly from the fold towards the loose edges and then wrung to spread the moisture throughout the towel. These prepared towels are then placed on the shelf within the towel steamer and will require approximately 20 minutes to heat throughout. Avoid over-wetting the towel prior to steaming as excessive moisture can scald your client. The case of the towel steamer can become very hot when in use; inform colleagues and clients to avoid touching this.

Remember: Do not undertake to use a razor, or any other sharp tool, near your client without first ensuring that there is adequate clear space around you to prevent other stylists obstructing the process.

Preparing your client

Gown your client, using the cutting cloth – a square sheet with a cut midway along one side. Ensure that your client's clothing is fully protected and draw the cloth up around the client's neck and tuck into the collar (see Figure 6.7).

Always use a clean gown for each of your clients; this will help to reduce the spread of infection or disorder from one client to the next. Place a clean light-coloured towel diagonally around the front of your client (see Figure 6.8), tucking the edges into the collar to protect your client's clothing. The use of a light-coloured towel will reflect light to the underside of the chin area.

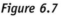

Figure 6.7

Figure 6.8

Discuss the shaving process with your client and establish the direction of beard growth by drawing your hands over the beard area. In one direction the beard will feel smooth and in the other the beard will feel at its roughest. The smooth feel will indicate the direction of growth. This

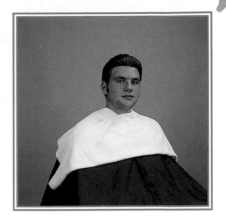

Remember: Ensure that your hands are clean and that any open sores or cuts on your hands are covered with a waterproof dressing.

direction is usually in a downward direction on the face. However, at times there are conflicting directions on the client's neck. Check the skin for any contra indications for shaving, including open cuts and abrasions, muscular swelling, contagious skin disorders and pustular eruptions. The location of any unusual feature/moles, etc, should be noted as they will be less apparent once the lather is in place.

Place a clean towel or tissue over the headrest of the chair, ask your client to support their own weight, recline the back of the chair to approximately 45° and then guide your client back onto the chair's back, adjusting the headrest to ensure that your client's neck area is not over stretched but so that it is exposed and lightly taught. Adjust the height of the chair so that your client's chin is at the level of your elbow.

Apply a steam towel to the beard area to help to soften the beard and cleanse the skin. Protecting your hands from the steam by using wooden tongs or a dry clean towel, remove a steam towel from the steamer, wring out any excess moisture, taking care not to allow the hot water to run onto your hands. Unwrap the towel, taking care that the steam given off does not scald your skin. A towel that is too hot may be held without causing pain to you by tossing the towel in your hands: this will also help it to cool more rapidly. With the towel still folded in half lengthways, stand at the back of the chair and put the towel close to the face.

Allow the face to become accustomed to the heat and then wrap the towels loosely around the face, taking care to ensure that all of the beard area is covered, but that the ears do not become covered, as they are sensitive to heat. Gentle pressure onto the towel around the beard area will increase the conduction of heat to the face. Remove the towel before it becomes cool and lather the beard area. The bristles of the lather brush should be preheated using hot water. Build up the lather in the lather bowl and then, using a rotary action, apply the lather to the beard area (see Figure 6.9).

Greater control of the lather may be achieved by gripping the handle and the tops of the bristles. While lathering the top lip, a finer spread of the brush may be achieved by fanning the bristles by pressing the finger into the base of the bristles (see Figure 6.10).

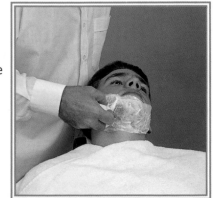

Figure 6.9

Lather will soften the beard and help to support the bristles away from the face. Ensure the face and lather is kept warm throughout the shaving process. To assist in softening the beard a further steam towel may be applied over the top of the lather. Remove this steam towel before it becomes cold and then re-lather the beard area. Once the lather is built up the shave may be carried out. A clean tissue or towel will be required on which to wipe the razor during the shaving process.

The shave

Hold the razor with the first two or three fingers and thumb on the shaft and the remainder on the tang. At all times the razor should be gripped firmly, with dry hands, but so that it may be manipulated from freehand and back hand positions.

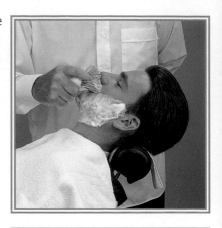

Figure 6.10

The movement of the razor is driven from the wrist. Stretch the skin taught, either behind or in front of the razor. Stretching the skin in front of the razor will give a more comfortable, less close shave, stretching behind the razor will give the reverse. If necessary remove lather from the face so that the skin may be stretched more effectively. Lie the razor on the skin, tilting the back of the razor away from the skin at approximately 30° and firmly but gently draw the razor across the beard. The shaving stroke must move the blade through the beard; avoid using a slicing action that will cut the skin. The shaving stroke is a smooth action extending only as far as the skin is taught. When shaving it is normal to shave positioned to the right-hand side of the client and at the back.

Remember: Never undertake a shaving stroke without holding the client's skin taught.

Should your client be cut while shaving apply a small amount of powdered Alum, a powdered styptic from a sterile dressing. Ferric chloride may be used as a liquid styptic. Never use an Alum stick, when it may be used on more than one client, as there may be a risk of spreading blood-related disorders.

Careful tensioning of the skin and correct movement of the razor considerably reduces risks of cutting your client. Take care when shaving over curved surfaces of the face, for example the chin, as it is easy to shave too close and cause short-term bleeding.

First-time over shave

In the main, the first-time over shave strokes follow the direction of beard growth.

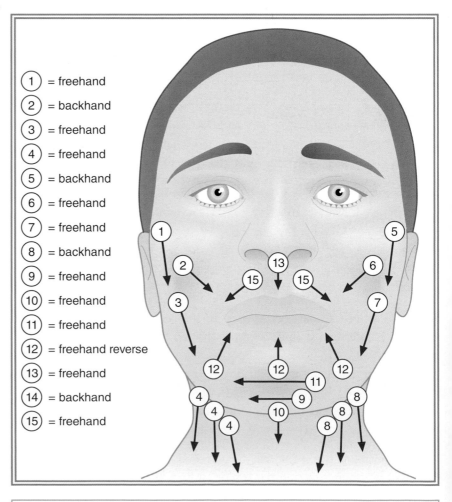

① = freehand
② = backhand
③ = freehand
④ = freehand
⑤ = backhand
⑥ = freehand
⑦ = freehand
⑧ = backhand
⑨ = freehand
⑩ = freehand
⑪ = freehand
⑫ = freehand reverse
⑬ = freehand
⑭ = backhand
⑮ = freehand

Figure 6.11 First-time over shaving strokes

Directions:

1 Standing at the side of your client, with your client's face turned away from you and starting at the sideburn lower edge stretch the skin and shave using a freehand movement, to the corner of the jaw (see Figure 6.12).

2 This is followed by a backhand movement across the cheek of your client. The exact start point for this movement will be determined by the extent of beard growth.

3 Stretching the skin upwards, shave freehand along the jawbone. Having stretched in this way, the jawbone will be free of hair once released.

4 Stretching both upwards and downwards, the under-jaw area is shaved using a freehand movement.

5 Turn your client's face towards you, and use a backhand movement to shave from the sideburn down to the corner of the jaw on the other side of the face (see Figure 6.13).

6 This is followed by a freehand movement across the cheek.

7 Stretch the skin upwards and shave, freehand, along the jawbone.

8 Standing slightly forward of your client stretch the under-jaw area, both upwards and downwards, and shave the area backhand. This area may require more than one stroke.

9 Move your client's face to a central position; apply fresh lather, if required.

10 Using a freehand movement and stretching either side of the chin and upwards, shave across the chin area. Take care not to shave too close as this may cause bleeding.

11 Standing slightly to the front of your client shave, freehand down the centre under-jaw area (see Figure 6.14).

12 Return to the side of your client and shave the upper chin area using a freehand movement,

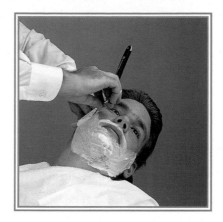

Figure 6.12

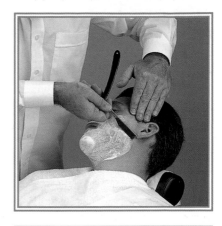

Figure 6.13

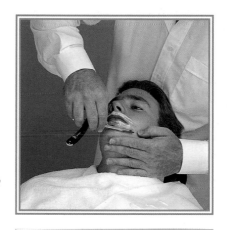

Figure 6.14

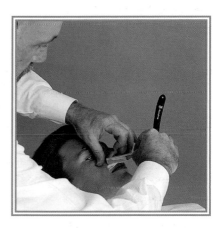

Figure 6.15

taking care not to draw the razor's point along the crease of the chin, below the lip.

13 Shave the area from the lip down to the crease of the skin, using a freehand movement, stretching the skin to either side of the mouth.

14 Shave the top lip, freehand down the centre of the top lip and then freehand one side and backhand of the far side of the top lip in an outward/downward direction (see Figure 6.15).

Remember: Do not leave an open razor lying unclosed when not in use as there is a risk of someone accidentally cutting themselves.

As the razor's blade becomes clogged or coated with lather and removed beard, wipe the blade by laying it flat on the tissue or towel, placed on your client's shoulder for this purpose, and drawing it across the towel with the razor's back leading. Never attempt a shaving movement when the razor's edge cannot be clearly seen.

Second-time over shave

These movements will remove the remaining beard giving a closer shave. The shaving stroke will, in the main, go against or across the direction of beard growth. More resistance to the razor will be experienced and firm but gentle movements must be used to overcome this without causing your client discomfort. Re-lather the beard, using fresh supplies of lather and hot water. Once the lather is built up the shave may commence.

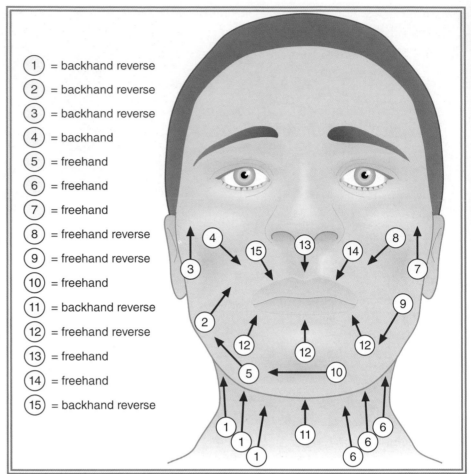

(1) = backhand reverse
(2) = backhand reverse
(3) = backhand reverse
(4) = backhand
(5) = freehand
(6) = freehand
(7) = freehand
(8) = freehand reverse
(9) = freehand reverse
(10) = freehand
(11) = backhand reverse
(12) = freehand reverse
(13) = freehand
(14) = freehand
(15) = backhand reverse

Figure 6.16 Second-time over shaving strokes

Directions:

1 Direct your client's face away from you, and starting from the hairline on the neck on the left side of your client, stretch down on the neck and shave upwards towards the jawbone using a reverse backhand stroke (see Figure 6.17).

2 The next reverse backhand stroke is used diagonally upwards across the jaw, stretching the skin in front of the razor, followed by a reverse backhand movement from the corner of the jawbone upwards towards the sideburn stretching downwards on the skin.

3 A backhand movement follows diagonally across the cheek area, as for the first-time over (see Figure 6.18).

4 Finally, on this side of the face, a backhand movement is used towards the chin along the jawbone in the chin area, stretching the skin back towards the corner of the jaw.

5 Move your client's face so it faces towards you. Standing slightly forward at the side of your client, starting at the hairline at the neck, use a reverse freehand stroke, stretching down on the neck (see Figure 6.19).

6 Move towards the back of your client, and reaching over him, use a reverse freehand movement shave from the corner of the jaw towards the sideburn, stretching the skin taught downwards behind the razor.

7 Moving back to the side of the client and using a freehand movement, shave across the cheek area, stretching the skin behind (see Figure 6.20). Stretching the skin upwards and back towards the client's ear, use a freehand movement to shave across the area of the jawbone.

8 With your client's face in the central position, and standing forward of the side of your client, use a reverse backhand movement to shave the central area under the chin, stretching downwards and out to each side.

9 Stretch the skin across the chin, pulling this area upwards as well, and shave across the chin using a freehand stroke.

10 Standing at the back of your client and reaching over him, stretch the chin area downwards and using a freehand movement shave the area between the crease of the chin and the bottom lip.

11 Move to the side of your client, shave the centre of the top lip in a downward direction, stretching the skin towards either side.

12 Stretch the nearest side of the top lip outwards and a backhand movement towards the middle. Stretch the furthest side of the top lip outwards and shave towards the centre using a freehand movement. Remove the towel or tissue used to wipe the razor free of lather and beard hair and dispose of it hygienically.

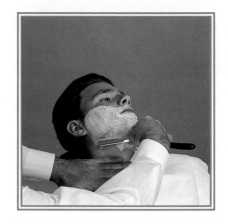

Figure 6.17

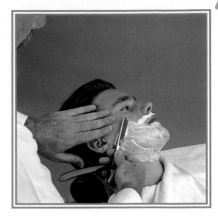

Figure 6.18

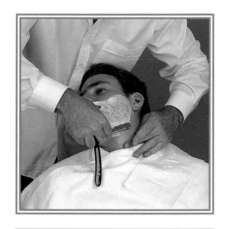

Figure 6.19

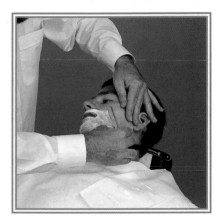

Figure 6.20

Following the completion of the shave a further hot towel is applied to your client's beard area. This should be removed from the face before cooling and then carefully wrapped around your hand and used to wipe any remaining lather from the face. Pay particular attention to the ear, nose and collar areas.

Remember: Do not attempt to shave the skin without a lubricant on the surface.

Having removed the hot towel, apply a cold towel to close the pores to prevent infection and aid retraction of the facial hair. Allow the cold towel to remain on the face for a few moments, using hand pressure to increase the conductivity of the cooling effect. A cold towel may be prepared in the same manner as a hot towel, using cold water and mild refrigeration to cool. This may be followed by the application of a mild astringent or aftershave, which will also close the pores and tighten the skin. When applying astringent, place a small amount on one hand, work this onto both hands and then using brisk, gentle slapping strokes apply this to the beard area, taking care not to be over-generous or to apply to the areas around the eyes.

Then fold a tissue onto your hand and use it to blot dry the surface of the skin, before applying un-perfumed talc, to soothe and remove shine from the skin. When applying talc to the face, place a small amount onto the hands and apply directly to the beard area or, using a talc puffer, shield your client's eyes and then apply directly to the face.

Remove the towel from your client and place in the laundry basket, and slowly raise the back of the hydraulic chair. A sudden movement may disorientate your client. Remove the linen gown protecting your client and, using a hand-held mirror, allow your client to check the surface of his skin.

For safety, before allowing your client to step from the hydraulic chair, ensure that it has been lowered and is locked into position.

These shaving movements have provided you with a basic structure to enable the shave to be completed. Provided the shave can be completed safely, without causing your client discomfort, effectively, these shaving strokes may be modified and adapted to suit your favoured mode of work and any individual characteristics of your client's beard area.

When shaving a very dark or heavy beard, an even closer shave may be achieved by sponge shaving. The technique follows the first two times over to shave against and across the direction of beard growth, drawing a warm moist sponge ahead of the razor. This action extends the hair out of the follicle, momentarily, allowing the hair to be cut closer before it retracts. Care must be taken as skin irritation may result from shaving too close, particularly on a face unaccustomed to wet shaving.

Immediately following the shave all material used must either be disposed of or washed and sterilised. Towels and gowns must be laundered, used tissue disposed of in a covered bin, the blade from the open razor must be removed (**if you are uncertain of how to remove the blade ask for guidance from your stylist or trainer**) and the used blade must be placed in a 'sharps box'.

> *Remember: The sharps box, when full, must be disposed of by hygienic incineration by a specialised company. Information about such companies may usually be obtained from an environmental health officer.*

For reasons of hygiene, a razor blade should be used on one client only. The casing of the razor should be washed, dried and placed in a liquid sterilising agent. Lather brushes must be washed and the bristles also placed in liquid sterilising fluid. All bowls, etc, must be cleaned and sterilised ready for their next use. All work surfaces should be wiped down using a proprietary surface cleaner.

Outline shaving

When shaving the outline of facial hair, use electrical clippers, inverted, to define the outline of the beard, moustache or sideburns. Moisten those areas of the beard to be removed, using lather, carefully applied so as not to affect the areas not to be shaved. Larger areas may have the lather applied using rotary movements with the lather brush, but smaller areas may require a stroking movement. The exact shaving strokes and their direction will be determined by the nature of the shape being outlined. Shaving strokes may have to be adapted to facilitate the clean and close removal of the unwanted beard.

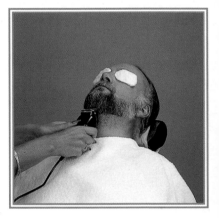

Figure 6.21 Inverted clipper to outline

Shaved hairlines

Nape hairlines that:

● must be clearly defined

● have excessively dark or vigorous hair growth or

● have very low points of growth

may be shaved using an open razor. All of the usual hygiene precautions must be observed. The area to be shaved is normally moistened with water and then, holding the skin taught, the hair is removed by shaving in the direction of hair growth. The skin, once dry, should be soothed by the application of fine talc. Take care not to shave too close and cause soreness or bleeding. Skin unaccustomed to this treatment will be particularly susceptible to soreness and irritation (see Figure 6.23).

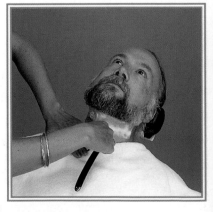

Figure 6.22 Shaving the outline

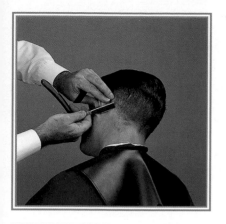

Figure 6.23 Shave side of nape hairline

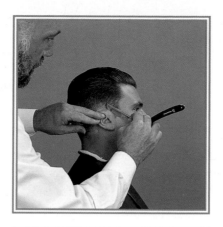

Figure 6.24 Shave above the ear

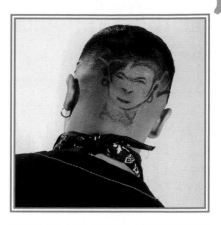

Figure 6.25 Decorative shaving in Afro-Caribbean hair

In the case of closely graduated sides, excessively low hairlines around the ears may be shaved, using short shaving strokes, taking care not to cut into the curve where the ear joins the scalp (see Figure 6.24).

In some Afro-Caribbean hair it is necessary to shave areas of the front hairline, when the hairline is particularly low or square. In very short Afro-Caribbean hair styles it may be necessary to shave parting areas, to give clear definition. A parting of approximately 3 mm width is shaved, having first used electric clippers to mark its position.

Remember: In all forms of shaving, high levels of hygiene are required at all times. All equipment must be thoroughly sterilised both before and after use.

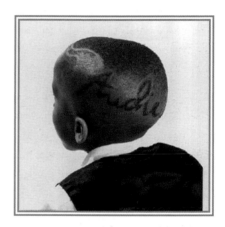

Figure 6.26 Decorative shaving in Afro-Caribbean hair

Review Questions

1 State two contraindications to carrying out a wet shave.

2 What steps should be taken should your client's skin be cut while shaving?

3 Suggest two reasons for tensioning the skin while shaving.

4 What benefit is gained by the use of steam towels?

5 What is the purpose of astringent lotions applied to the skin following a wet shave?

6 In what directions would the first-time over shaving strokes follow?

7 How should sharps be disposed of?

8 What is the benefit of shaving the nape hairline?

Additional information

Useful websites

Website Addresses	Content
www.habia.org.uk	Hairdressing and Beauty Industry Authority. Downloads available including references to other websites
www.bbc-safety.co.uk	Free advice on health and safety
www.lookfantastic.com	Professional hairdressing products and advice
www.laurandp.co.uk	Educational publications for development of professional hairdressing
www.scott999.fsnet.co.uk	Hairdressing product information
www.keratin.com	Hair and scalp disorders
www.trichologists.org.uk	Institute of Trichologists

The evidence from the activities below will cover the Underpinning Knowledge for the Technical Certificate for Advanced Modern Apprenticeships. You will need to take the external test and carry out the practical activities. (see City and Guilds Diploma Hairdressing 6915/6913).

Activity

Outcome 1

- Describe the correct use of shaving tools and equipment and the effects they have.
- Explain how to maintain and prepare shaving equipment.
- Describe the different effects created by different shaving techniques.
- State what factors need to be considered when providing shaving services.
- Describe the safety considerations that must be taken into account when providing shaving services.
- List the range of products available and state the effects they have on the skin.
- List the problems that may occur during shaving services and state how to resolve them.
- State the importance of using personal protective equipment.
- Explain why skin needs to be tensioned during shaving.
- State the importance of not shaving too close.
- State the importance of considering the density and direction of the hair growth during shaving.
- State the reasons for and the effects of using hot and cool towels.
- State when shaving services should not be carried out.
- Explain how to dispose of sharps safely.

- List the methods of sterilisation and sanitation available and state which are suitable for use in the barbers' shop.

- State the importance of avoiding cross infections and infestations.

- Outline the health and safety legislation for:

  The Health and Safety at Work Act (1974).

  The Management of Health and Safety at Work Regulations (1992).

  The Personal Protective Equipment at Work Regulations (1992).

  The Provision and Use of Work Equipment at Work Regulations (1992).

  The Control of Substances Hazardous to Health Regulations (1992).

  The Electricity at Work Regulations (1989).

  The Workplace (Health, Safety and Welfare) Regulations (1992).

  Local Byelaws.

  and explain how they affect you and your salon.

7 UNIT H20 DESIGN AND CREATE A RANGE OF FACIAL HAIR SHAPES

1 Maintain effective and safe methods of working when cutting facial hair

2 Create a range of facial hair shapes

CHAPTER CONTENTS

- *Client Preparation*
- *Barbering Tools*
- *Cutting Facial Hair*
- *Beard Shaping*
- *Moustache Shaping*
- *Sideburn Trimming*

- *The Complete Service*
- *Further Study*
- *Review Questions*
- *Additional Information*
- *Activity*

Introduction

Barbering invariably involves attention to facial hair, whether it is to level sideburns or, at the other extreme, to shape a full beard and moustache. Facial hair, just as scalp hair, may be used to enhance the wearer's appearance. It can alter the apparent shape of the face, drawing attention to or reducing the effects of a range of facial features.

Facial hair must be considered part of the total look of your client. Most men have hair growth on the face, some choosing to grow this and others preferring to be cleanly shaved. As there is a presence of facial hair the barber must be able to work with this. Even the cleanly shaved face will require those areas of the hairstyle which join to the beard area to be cut and cleanly lined.

To ignore the total appearance of your client when barbering would be a great error. Having styled the hair on the scalp, neglect of any facial hair, subject to your client's agreement, would equate to failure to complete a hairstyle.

Remember, shaping facial hair evenly and cleanly is something that your client will find difficult to undertake, as they can only observe the beard from one angle. You have the advantage of being able to offer the client something that they are not able to undertake themselves to the same level of proficiency.

Client preparation

Seating your client

Barbering skills usually require the use of a hydraulically operated chair for the client (see Figure 7.1).

This allows you, the barber, to raise or lower and position your client at a height and

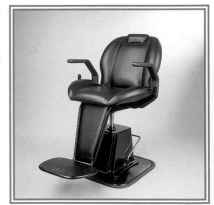

Figure 7.1 Hydraulically operated chair

angle that allows you easy and comfortable access to all areas of the scalp and face when cutting, no matter what the physical height of your client. To shape facial hair your client is best slightly reclined. This makes the chin area of the face more accessible. A chair with this facility is a great advantage for the barber and for your client's comfort.

Always ensure that the hydraulic chair is clean and free from hair cuttings. Lower the chair to its lowest position – at this height the chair is most stable and least likely to tip or move. In the case of a manual hydraulic chair this may be done by depressing the foot pump and holding it down while the chair falls. Some pressure on the chair may be required to encourage it on its downward journey. Once at the desired height, pull the foot lever upwards, by placing a foot beneath and jerking upwards. This locks the chair in position and prevents it from revolving. Electronically operated chairs are available and the manufacturer's directions for use should be followed.

Remember: If you are uncertain of the safe working of the chair ask for guidance from your line manager or trainer.

Once your client is seated, the chair may be adjusted to a height to suit your work.

Client consultation

Discuss with your client the treatment to be given. Listen to you client. Additional information about client consultation can be found in Chapter 3.

When consulting with your client you should remember that there will be a number of reasons why men keep their facial hair. It may be used purely as a fashion tool, enabling the wearer to produce a particular look for the moment, or to cover facial blemishes or scarring. The apparent shape of the face can be altered considerably by the use of facial hair and in discussing and carrying out a beard or moustache trim it is essential that you identify the requirements of your client before proceeding.

Gowning your client

The cutting cloth or cape is usually a square or rectangular shape with a slit in the middle of one side. This slit is to fit your client's neck, being tucked into the client's collar. Ensure that the gown covers your client's clothing. When cutting, a strand of cotton wool is tucked between the gown and the neck. This forms a seal to prevent hair clippings from passing down the neck. A cutting collar may also be used to hold the gown in place while cutting.

Personal hygiene

It is particularly important to be aware of your own personal hygiene as you will be working very close to your client. Body odour can be offensive to your client as can liberal use of strong-smelling perfume and cologne. Oral hygiene is also very important. Breath smelling of strong-tasting foods, cigarette smoke or the effects of halitosis or decaying teeth can be unpleasant to your client. Keep your breath fresh, particularly when working closely with your client or colleagues.

Barbering tools

All tools should be of good quality and hygienically clean. At the work station there must be a method of easily sterilising tools between clients. Usually a second set of tools is required, so that sterilising may take place while you continue to work.

Scissors

Scissors should be of a professional standard. They are made from a good quality steel that are rust free and can be sterilised easily. They come in various lengths, weight and quality. Scissors vary from 10–18 cm in length. Most barbers prefer longer length (around 15 cm) for scissor over comb techniques, depending on the size of your hand or the job you need to carry out. Both left- and right-handed scissors are available.

The correct scissor hold is important to ensure you can cut as close to the skin as possible.

You need to maintain them by following manufacturer's instructions and sharpen them regularly to prevent causing any discomfort to the client.

Combs

A range of combs is required. Some should have both fine- and coarse-set teeth and be a range of sizes. Fine, flexible-backed combs can flex and fit against the contour of the face and neck. This is particularly necessary when close graduating. Rigid-backed combs are able to cope with strong hair.

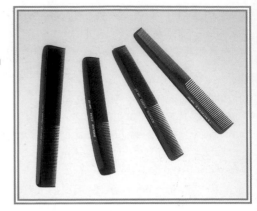

Figure 7.2 Barbering combs

Hair clippers

There are a number of clippers and trimmers available. Make sure you read the manufacturer's instructions for use and care whilst using. Clippers can be hand operated or electric. These act as shears, cutting the hair. They must be oiled regularly and cleaned after each client.

Hand clippers tend not to be used so much these days, especially where electricity is available. Electric clippers are either charged by electricity or re-chargeable batteries. This type of clipper is preferred due to the power, accuracy and convenience when compared to hand clippers.

Clippers must be of good quality for professional use and should be sterilised after each use. Follow manufacturer's instructions for maintainence.

Oiling the heads of the clippers regularly is required and making sure the heads are balanced correctly.

The correct power supply should be used and safety precautions taken when using electrical appliances, e.g. use on dry hair, make sure your hands are also dry when in use. Beware of trailing flexes and loose wires, etc. Keep them out of reach from children. Disconnect them after use. Change the heads when needed and oil regularly. Make sure if using the clipper attachments that they are fixed on securely and are not broken. A number of ranges of electric hair clippers have graders that may be attached. The grader sets a gap between the face and the cutting blade, enabling a consistent length of hair to be cut. These graders vary in size, the smallest (producing the closest cut being 'number 1' progressing to the larger 'number 8'). Graders are available that have a graduating effect on the hair, if the clipper is inserted sideways into the hair.

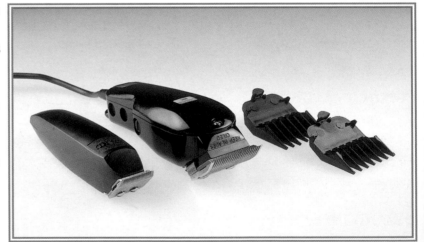

Figure 7.3 Hair clippers

Read the Electricity at Work Act. Maintenance of the clippers is your responsibility so make sure you work safely and eliminate any risk to yourself or clients. More information is provided in Chapter 1.

Razors

See Unit H18 for further information.

Neck brushes

Neck brushes should be of good quality and soft so that they are comfortable for the client when brushing away the hair from the skin. Again these need to be sterilised after use and kept in good condition. Follow manufacturer's instructions for care details

Talcum powder dispensers

These come in various shapes and sizes and are professional products. Normally the refillable puffer containers are made from a good quality rubber with small holes on the top so that the talcum powder comes out evenly. These should be wiped down and kept free from dirt and hair.

Cutting facial hair

Please read Units G1, G6, G9 and H18 prior to this unit, relating to health and safety, consultation, aftercare and shaving.

To carry out a hair cut and neglect the extremities on the face, for example the base of the sideburns, or to neglect the concept of the total look would be an error. To present the male client, the barber must consider the total appearance of the head and face together. When cutting and shaping facial hair, remember that you are producing a three-dimensional shape onto the face. The face is made of irregular shapes over which you must work.

Consultation

1. What does your client want?
2. Does he want a beard or moustache, etc?
3. Does he have any signs of broken skin, abnormalities, etc?
4. Does he have anything that may limit you carrying out the service, e.g. contagious disorders?
5. Is the beard hair fine, medium or coarse?
6. Is the beard growth dense or sparse?
7. Is the density of the beard growth uneven around the face?
8. Pay attention to the client's face shape.
9. Consider the total look, e.g. existing hair cut.
10. Look at the facial features, e.g. breadth and depth of the chin and jaw lines (see Unit H18).
11. Look at the hair growth patterns.
12. Look at the texture of the hair.
13. Look at the shape of the face – round, square, oblong, small, long, etc.
14. Look for scars, moles, dimples and bald spots, etc.

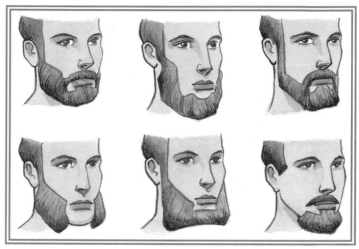

Figure 7.4 A range of beard shapes

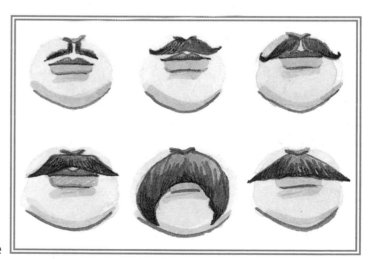

Figure 7.5 A range of moustache shapes

Remember: Discuss, fully, with your client the desired shape and effect required from the facial hair before starting to shape.

Facial hair may be shaped using:

- haircutting scissors and/or electric clippers, over a comb, to shape
- freehand cutting using the scissors, to cut outlines or shape small areas
- inverted clippers, to outline the perimeter shape
- razor, to remove unwanted facial hair around the perimeter or the shape.

Beard shaping

Client preparation

Following the consultation, place a light-coloured towel diagonally across your client's chest, tuck in one side of the collar, then fold the towel to enclose the other side of the neck. The light towel will reflect light up under the chin area, as well as providing a surface against which to check the profile of the beard. Ensure that there is no gap between the neck and towel.

Recline the back of the chair slightly and then protect your client's eyes from hair clippings by either placing moist cotton wool pads or by draping a small hand towel across the eyes. A clean tissue should be placed across any head rest to reduce the risk of infection from one client to the next.

Comb the beard to remove tangles, in some cases it may be necessary to lightly moisten the beard to soften dressings. Take care not to over-moisten, particularly if the use of electric clippers is to follow. While combing the beard, check for any strong or uneven growth patterns that may impact upon the finished shape. Many strong patterns have a greater impact upon the beard as it is reduced in length.

Outline shaping

Comb the hair thoroughly to lift it from the face. Check for any areas of thinness that may require specialist attention. Using the inverted clipper define the outline shape, by pressing the cutting edge into the beard at the required point (see Figure 7.6).

Using the clipper, remove the excess hair from this area.

Shave this area free of hair using the techniques described in Chapter 6.

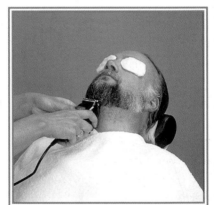

Figure 7.6 Outline shaping

> *Remember: If your client wears a full beard, it may not be necessary to define the outline. Consult with your client.*

Shaping the bulk of the beard

Comb the hair to allow it to lie in its natural position. Insert the teeth of the comb at the position of the required cut and then using either scissor or clippers cut the hair to the level of the comb (see Figure 7.7).

Your choice of cutting tool will depend upon:

- personal preference
- coarseness and thickness of the beard, with a coarser beard being easier cut using electric clippers
- shape to be produced.

Move the comb slowly over the beard shape describing the shape required, and cut at

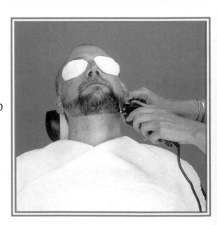

Figure 7.7 Shaping the bulk of the beard

this point. Take care to observe the profile and balance of the shape being produced, using the mirror and by checking against the light surface of the protective towel.

Shaping normally commences at the side of the beard, where it joins the hairstyle on the scalp. In most cases the two should flow together. The shape produced on the face may not be that of the face and therefore care must be taken to hold the comb in the correct position, which follows the outline shape. Take care not to shape too short in areas of thin hair; the area where the moustache joins the beard is often thinner. The area beneath the chin will often appear shorter when the head is reclined and once upright will appear still quite full. Be careful not to take away corners or points if they are required in the finished shape.

Remove clippings from the neck and avoid a build-up of clippings that may become trapped between the skin and your client's clothing.

The line along the top lip of the moustache is cut using either the inverted clipper or by freehand cutting using scissors.

Completion

Comb the facial hair fully to remove any loose hair clippings. Remove any protective pads from over your client's eyes and use a tissue to wipe any clippings from the face. Dust the clippings from your client's neck area and remove the protective towel, taking care not to allow clippings to pass down the collar. Gently raise the back of your client's chair, and then pass him a hand mirror with which to view the beard.

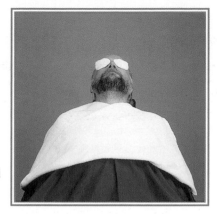

Figure 7.8 Client with cotton wool pads on eyes

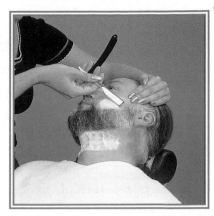

Figure 7.9 Outline shaving

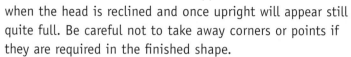

Remember: When cutting very curly facial hair, allowance should be made for the hair to spring back into place, therefore producing a closer shape.

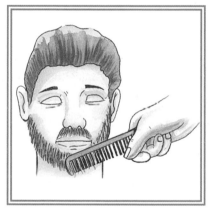

Figure 7.10 Combing beard

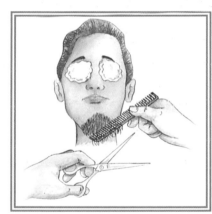

Figure 7.11 Trimming goatee beard

Moustache shaping

When trimming the moustache, it may not be necessary to gown your client with a light-coloured towel, as the moustache will be viewed against the face, not the towel. Having reclined the chair, using the clippers, outline the shape of the moustache area. The shaping may be carried out above the moustache or between the moustache and lips. This area may then be shaved free of hair.

Many moustaches have hair that is shaped to extend past the area of actual growth. Take care not to remove this, comb the hair into place and cut the required length over the lip. If the hair projects onto the lip, scissors should be used, taking care to use the free hand to steady the blades.

Check for balance and evenness of length. Beards may require the application of dressing to produce the required result, moustache wax may be applied to stiffen the hair to enable 'handle bar' effects to be achieved.

Sideburn trimming

For all barbering the finished length of the sideburns must be checked, adjusted and made even. Sideburns that may have appeared quite flat before the haircut will need to be cut in proportion when the scalp hair has been trimmed. The barber must be able to offer this service.

Following consultation with your client, and cutting using either scissor or clipper over the comb, reduce the bulk of the sideburns. Invert the clipper to cut the lower edge (see Figure 7.12), using the mirror to check balance. Use your thumbs to indicate the base level of the sideburn, and view this in the mirror to check for evenness. Remember that facial features may not always be even on each side of the face. Having cut the lower line it may be necessary to soften the line with slight graduation.

Sideburns may be used to add shape to the face and may require consideration not only in their lower line but also in the profile shape. When removing the bulk, use the comb over which you are cutting, to determine the profile shape being achieved. Use the mirror to monitor the progress in the shape. The outline shape of the sideburn may require shaving once complete.

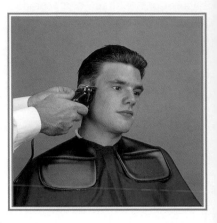

Figure 7.12 Using inverted clipper on sideburns

The complete service

As the professional barber, remember your client's total look. Be prepared to offer to remove hair from the ears, using the clippers or with extreme care using the points of the scissors. Be prepared to trim eyebrows and to clean even lines around your hairstyle. This includes the bases of sideburns, around the ears of very short hairstyles and the nape both behind the ears and on the neck. Remember your client does not always wear a high-collared shirt. There will be times when t-shirts may be worn, and therefore neck hair may need to be removed to a lower level.

Further study

There are a number of beard and moustache shapes, most of which have names to describe them. Find out more about these and learn those more usual ones.

Review Questions

1 *How should the electric clipper be used to outline a beard?*

2 *In what position should the hydraulic chair be when the client is invited to sit?*

3 *Why is a light-coloured towel used when beard trimming?*

4 *What is the largest size clipper grader available?*

5 *Why is a tissue placed on the chair's headrest while trimming the beard?*

6 *When beard trimming, will the area beneath the chin appear longer or shorter when the head is upright?*

7 *Why is the scissor over comb used in preference to holding the hair with the fingers?*

8 *Is the razor used on wet or dry surfaces?*

Additional information

Useful websites

Website Addresses	Content
www.habia.org.uk	Hairdressing and Beauty Industry Authority. Downloads available including references to other websites
www.bbc.safety.co.uk	Free advice on diseases in hairdressing
www.lookfantastic.com	Professional hairdressing products and advice
www.laurandp.co.uk	Educational publications for development of professional hairdressing
www.scott999.fsnet.co.uk	Hairdressing product information
www.trichologists.org.uk	Institute of Trichologists

The evidence from the activities below will cover the Underpinning Knowledge for the Technical Certificate for Advanced Modern Apprenticeships. You will need to take the external test and carry out the practical activities (see City and Guilds Diploma Hairdressing 6915/6913).

ACTIVITY

Outcome 1

- *Describe the correct use of cutting equipment.*
- *Explain how to maintain cutting equipment.*
- *Describe the effects created by different cutting techniques.*
- *State why factors need to be considered when cutting beards and moustaches.*
- *Explain the safety considerations that must be taken into account when cutting beards and moustaches.*
- *Describe the range of traditional and current fashion beard and moustache looks.*
- *Explain how to make sure that outline shapes are cut level.*
- *Explain how to dispose of sharps safely.*
- *Explain how to check and look after electrical equipment for safe use.*

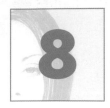

8 UNIT H21 CREATE A VARIETY OF LOOKS USING BARBERING TECHNIQUES

1 Maintain effective and safe methods of working when cutting hair

2 Create a variety of looks for men

CHAPTER CONTENTS

- Preparation
- Barbering Tools
- The Barbered Haircut
- Men's Haircutting
- Teenagers' Haircutting
- Children's Haircutting
- Consultation Points
- The Graduated Cut 'Classic Style' – Traditional

- The Sculptured Haircut – 'Artistic'
- Drying the Style
- Style Variations
- Review Questions
- Additional Information
- Activity

Introduction

Those traditional skills closely associated with men's hairdressing include close graduation and sculptured looks, facial hair work and facial hair removal. Traditionally the shapes produced in men's hair are square and much sharper than those usually associated with other forms of hairstyling. They are produced using techniques that facilitate the easy manipulation of short hair using the comb combined with clippers or scissors, either on the scalp or face.

This chapter will provide the essential knowledge necessary for the understanding of barbering skills and will provide you with guidance in the procedures and techniques used within this skill.

Preparation

Seating your client

Barbering skills usually require the use of a hydraulically operated chair for the client (see Figure 7.1).

Ensure that the back of the chair is in an upright position and, if you are about to cut the scalp hair, remove the headrest. If attached its location can often prevent you from working with ease in the nape area of your client's hairstyle. Once your client is seated, the chair may be adjusted to a height to suit your work. More information is provided in Unit H19.

Client consultation

Discuss with your client the treatment to be given. Listen to the client. Additional information about client consultation is contained within Unit G9.

Gowning your client

The cutting cloth or cape is usually a square or rectangular shape with a slit in the middle of one side. This slit is to fit your client's neck, being tucked into the client's collar. Ensure that the gown covers your client's clothing. When cutting, a strand of cotton wool is tucked between the gown and the neck. This forms a seal to prevent hair clippings from passing down the neck. A cutting collar may also be used to hold the gown in place while cutting.

Barbering tools

All tools should be of good quality and hygienically clean. At the work station there must be a method of easily sterilising tools between clients. Usually a second set of tools is required, so that sterilisation can take place while you continue to work.

Scissors

Scissors should be of a professional standard. They are made from a good quality steel that is rust free and can be sterilised easily. Thinning scissors have serrated edges to the blades that can vary in length and thickness. This determines the volume of hair removal and how fine the taper is. More information is provided in Unit H19.

Combs

Combs set with even teeth may be used when producing flat surfaces on the hair. Combs with a range of coarse and fine teeth may be used when producing longer as well as closely graduated looks. Fine, flexible combs allow the back of the comb to flex against the scalp, following the contours. These enable a very close graduation to be achieved. Fashion styling effects may be achieved using specialist styling combs. More information is provided in Unit H19.

Hair clippers

There are a number of clippers and trimmers on the market so make sure you read the manufacturer's instructions for use and care whilst using. More information is provided in Unit H19.

Brushes

A range of brushes is required. Closely set bristle brushes are able to pick up and hold short graduated hair. Coarser set bristles may produce textured effects in completed dressings. A neck brush will be required, to dust hair clipping from your client's skin.

The barbered haircut

Two types of haircuts are covered within this section. One has a closely graduated natural hairline effect and the other requires a more sculptured artistic look, the latter being more closely associated with traditional men's hairdressing competition looks.

Both haircuts may be carried out on wet or dry hair. Cutting hair when wet will give more control and reduce hair clippings flying over yourself and your client.

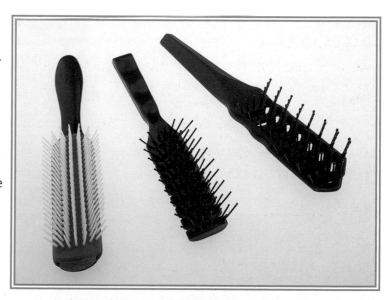

Figure 8.1 Blow drying brushes

Please read Unit G1 regarding health and safety especially relating to sterilisation of tools and equipment, reducing risk, and disposing of sharps.

Take care of tools appropriately. There is a lot of information in Units H18 and H19 relating to this.

Unit H26 covers cutting for women but a lot of this information relates to men's haircutting on all the cutting techniques, e.g. rounded layers, square layers, point cutting, texturising, club cutting, etc. Men's haircuts are usually a lot shorter but the techniques are similar, especially for fashion cutting.

The textures of the hair and growth patterns are very important as the same haircut on two different textures will give a completely different look. You need to be very aware. There are different types of hair, for example straight, curly, wavy, Caucasian, Asian, Afro-Caribbean (see Unit G9).

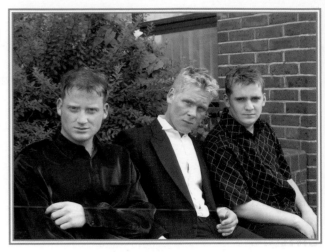

Figure 8.2 Barbered haircuts

Hairlines can differ greatly, e.g. high hairline, low hairlines, whorls and uneven hairlines. This can be critical when cutting hair very short and the appropriate techniques will need to be used. You should already have a basic understanding of hair types and cutting techniques and should have gained experience regarding what works well. At this point you need to take the consultation much further by matching this experience and continually updating your skills to provide a professional service for traditional and fashionable looks.

You can do this by combining cutting techniques to produce the looks seen on the catwalks in the media, etc. You can also design your own creative images by taking this a step further. Read Unit H23 if you feel you would like to explore and develop your own creative ability.

Gown your client with a cutting cloth, cotton wool and a cutting shoulder cape (see Figure 8.3).

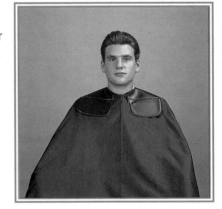

Figure 8.3 Client gowned for cut

Following a consultation check the hair for any strong hair growth patterns, degree of curl, length and texture. The hair should be pre-shampooed if required: this is recommended. You should be aware that within a barbering context there will be a number of clients who do not wish to have their hair shampooed and it may be necessary to lightly spray the hair with water to achieve effective control. Avoid wetting the hair when cutting using electrical clippers. Remember the hair stretches when wet and shrinks when dry due to its elastic structure. You may need to thin the hair more once it has dried, especially if it is thick and wavy. Leave the hair longer when wet to allow for the hair to shrink especially if it is fine or curly.

Men's haircutting

The hair is terminal and can be very coarse and strong. It can also be very fine and thin depending on heredity, physical well-being and environmental factors. Men who start losing hair can become very sensitive and need to be dealt with tactfully and diplomatically. They have grown with their hair and can tell you a lot in terms of what will and won't work, so listen carefully. They might not always be right and it's up to you to encourage them to try something new if you feel it would look better. Gain their trust first then start to make some suggestions. Discuss with them in detail.

In general, men tend to go for traditional and fashionable looks.

Teenagers' haircutting

Once past puberty hair is called terminal hair. However, some teenagers can still have vellus hair which is fine and soft. The areas around the sideburns can still be very patchy and it is easy to cut off too much. Be careful around this area as teenage boys can become very sensitive if you take away their only bit of hair. Some teenagers can have very strong hair growth around the face shape and the sideburns will need shaping as in men's haircutting.

Usually at this stage teenagers like to feel part of the crowd and go for fashionable looks. This does vary greatly in terms of how fashionable and what image they want to reflect. Showing haircuts from magazines can be very useful to help them describe what they want and for you to suggest what is needed. Today there is such a wide variety of styles to choose from – shaven looks, graded looks, texturised, spiky, long, medium and short styles. Make sure you assess the length and type of hair before confirming you are able to do what is requested.

Children's haircutting

Children's hair tends to be softer and finer and is called vellus hair. The hair can also be thick or fine. You need to be careful when cutting children's hair especially when using the clippers as they can become fidgety. Be very careful not to leave tools and equipment within their reach. Make sure you agree with their parents as to what hairstyle is required and try not to keep them sitting for too long. Remember safety first and reduce any potential risk. Have some photographs of children's hairstyles available to help you and your client to decide.

Consultation points

Below are some points to help you through the consultation prior to cutting men's, teenagers' and children's hair.

- What hairstyle does the client want?
- Does he have any hair or scalp problems, or abnormalities?
- Does he have anything that may limit you carrying out the cut, e.g. anything contagious?
- Is the hair fine, medium or coarse?
- Is the hair growth dense or sparse?
- Is the hair growth uneven, e.g. does the hair recede?
- Does he have a beard or moustache that the haircut needs to compliment?
- Look at his sideburns. What length, shape and thinness/thickness does he require and how will you blend them?
- Does he have sparse areas in the sideburn shape?
- What outline does he require, e.g. round, square or v-shape?
- Pay attention to the client's face shape.
- Consider the total look, e.g. clothing style, facial hair, jewellery.
- Look at the facial features, e.g. breadth and depth of the chin and jaw lines.
- Look at the hair growth patterns.
- Look at the texture of the hair.
- Look at the shape of the face, e.g. round, square, oblong, small, long, etc.
- Look for scars, moles and bald spots.
- What personalising techniques will you use, e.g. texturising, pointing, thinning, or scissor over comb?
- What tools and equipment will you use?
- Make sure you agree on the haircut to be carried out.
- Show some photographs of men's hairstyles to help the client to choose his hair style.

● Recommend the correct products to use to achieve the finished result.

● Read through Units G1, G6, G9 and H8.

The graduated cut 'classic style' – traditional

This style is the classic closely graduated hairstyle, having a nape hairline that blends with the neck. The exact point that the haircut ends and the neck line begins is almost indiscernible.

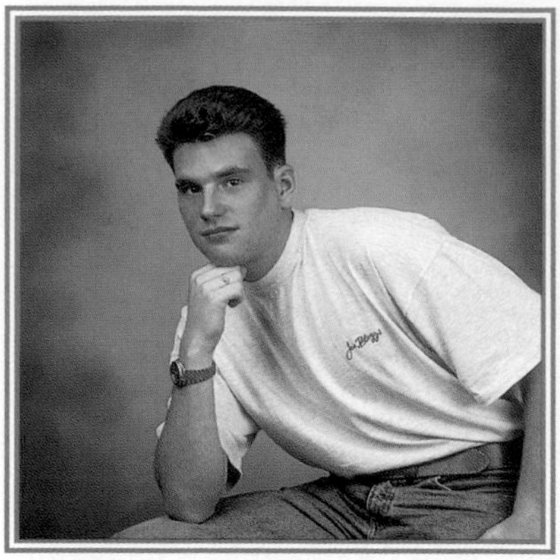

Figure 8.4 Finished graduated haircut

Directions:

1 *With the hair moist or almost dry and starting at the centre back of the head slide the points of the scissors through the hair, close to the scalp at the outermost point of the occipital bone.*

2 *Lift the hair section and place onto the comb.*

3 *Lift the mesh out from the head at 90 degrees and cut to the required length. Note the position of the back of the comb in the hair.*

4 *Moving down the head slide the scissor through the hair, at the scalp, 0.5 cm beneath the previous section and place the hair onto the comb.*

5 *Lift the mesh of hair, together with the previously cut mesh, out from the head, at less than 90 degrees and cut to the same length as the previously cut hair. The lower the hair section is held the shorter the subsequent section of hair cut will be. Therefore you control the hairstyle.*

6 *At all times the section for the meshes should be taken at right angles to the hairline.*

7 *Continue down the head in the same manner until the hairline is reached. Then at the hairline insert a fine toothed, flexible backed comb and, pressing it against the scalp, with the comb teeth projecting slightly out, move the comb upwards and gradually out from the scalp, cutting with the scissors continuously as you go. A steady and continuous movement of the comb, coupled with a continuous cutting action, will ensure a smooth, even graduation without steps or cutting marks.*

8 *Move to a point adjacent to the first section cut and repeat the process. Always include a small section of the adjacent cut mesh of hair as a guide to the cut line.*

9 *Continue around to the side of the head in this manner; remember that the sections and your comb must follow the design or hairline. Ensure that your comb is parallel to the hairline at all times.*

10 *Once the front hairline is reached, return to the centre back and commence the movement to the other side of the head.*

11 *Once the lower areas of the hair have been cut, the top should be addressed. Starting at the front hairline take sections of hair, 1 cm in depth, and hold out at 90 degrees and cut to the same length as the very first cut at the occipital bone.*

12 *Taking small sections continue from the front in columns, taking meshes of hair at 90 degrees and cutting to the same length as the previous sections until the occipital area is reached. Always include a small mesh of already cut hair, within the mesh, to act as a guide to the cutting line.*

13 *Having completed this with one row, start at the front hairline and work back with another row, and continue to do so until the top area of the hair is cut and blends with the graduated side areas. The top area will now have a uniform layer and the side and back a graduation.*

14 It may be necessary to taper the hair where the uniform layer meets the graduation, on the curve of the head, as within this area there will be considerable volume of hair.

15 For a truly graduated hairline the nape area must be closely blended. This may be achieved by the use of electric clippers. Using clippers with a variable cut setting, set for the longest cut and slide the clipper up the neck into the hairline, gradually pivoting the cutting blade away from the hair. Repeat this several times, each time reducing the gauge of the cut and the distance up the hairline that this progresses.

This task may also be carried out using the very fine teeth of the comb, pushing the comb flat to the neck, gradually tilting the teeth and moving the comb away from the neck and scalp and cutting the hair that projects through the comb's teeth as you go.

Remember: For your client's comfort, hair clipping should be dusted from the neck area regularly.

A truly graduated haircut will have a blend with no obvious demarcation lines or 'steps'.

The exact end of the hairstyle and beginning of the neck area will be almost undetectable. When a very short-haired result is required, particularly on dark hair, it may be necessary to shave away the hair from just above the ear, behind the ear (on the hairline) and the nape (without producing a definite hairline).

Details of outline shaving are included in Unit H19.

The sculptured haircut – 'artistic'

This cut is generally less graduated than the previous, being slightly more of a uniform layer. The hair is often cut wet, starting with the hair being thinned. This may be achieved by using thinning scissors or a razor.

Remember: Consult your client throughout the cutting process to check for satisfaction and to consult on shape and length.

Thinning scissors

Systematically work over the head cutting each mesh of hair using the thinning scissor. Avoid over-thinning the front hairline, paring area and the crown. To avoid a line of demarcation, use the thinning scissor lightly along the entire length of the hair rather than just the once.

When used on wet hair thinning scissors will remove more volume than when used on dry.

Razor thinning

The razor should be used only on wet or moist hair. Having checked the scalp for any protrusions, section the hair off starting at the nape, using sections 1 cm deep. Use a co-ordinated comb and razor action (see Figure 8.5).

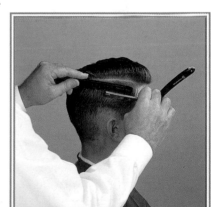

Figure 8.5 Razor cutting

Draw the razor along the last three-quarters of the hair's length in the direction in which the hair will lie. Complete this section by section throughout the haircut, taking care in areas where the head curves as these areas may be over-thinned if a sharp razor is used. The hair of the top of the head is normally combed forward and thinned in this manner and the side is combed forward so as to avoid your client's ears.

Remember: Before razor-thinning the hair, always check the scalp for any lumps or bumps.

The curl of over curly hair may be reduced by thinning the ends of the meshes in this manner and very straight hair may be styled more easily.

Layering

The actual haircut may commence at any part of the head. This is often the nape or front hairline, usually at the shortest point. Take a mesh of hair, comb this at 90 degrees out from the head and cut to the required length. Continue over the head in this manner, using a previously cut mesh of hair as a guide to the cutting line. Remember that a square or angular shape is required for men, so do not round off corners at the side curvature of the head or at the crown.

Section the hair using horizontal sections across the top of the head to the widest part of the head shape, leaving the corners on. When working the side sections use vertical sections to blend the hair length from the widest point down into the sides and the nape area, which has been previously cut short by clippers or scissor over comb technique, grading the hair from long to shorter. You will need to cross check to ensure that the hair cut is even, thus preventing steps in the hair. Ensure that you work with the growth patterns and texture to achieve the desired result.

Once the layering is complete, the hair may need additional thinning to compensate for hair that has been removed by the cut.

The hair must now be outlined. This is done by moistening the hair and combing down, using the back of the comb to flatten the hair against the skin. The scissors or inverted clipper may then be used to cut the outline shape. Remember most men's hairstyles have square-shaped necklines. These are either definite square shapes, the line behind the ear being cut in a downward line using the scissors, pointed from the ear down to the nape and then squared across the nape using scissors or inverted clippers, or downward lines either side of the nape with a graduated neckline.

A 'Boston' neckline is a heavy abrupt napeline across the back of the nape, curving slightly to accentuate the width.

You may want the hair to stand up, e.g. flat top or spiky. Further personalising techniques can be used by point cutting, etc (see Unit H26).

You may wish to leave the top layers much longer, therefore you will need to use cutting angles of 45 degrees to allow for a much steeper graduation and diagonal sections. To do this you will want to use a graduation technique by taking note of the following steps.

It is important to feel the head shape so that you can compensate the haircut technique for flat occipital bones, or uneven head shapes, scars, etc. It is all about distribution of weight to make the hairstyle complement the client.

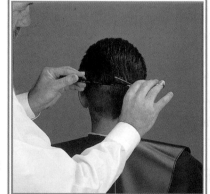

The texture of the hair will also give different results, e.g. coarse hair may stick up if it is cut too short, whereas fine hair can fall flat if left too long. Hair shrinks when it is dry up to 30% depending on the elasticity.

Figure 8.5a Graduated hair cut

Hairlines can be left soft or hard. Shapes can be cut in; they can be square or rounded depending on the client's wishes. Some hairlines are uneven or grow in different directions. Using the comb flat and turning it clockwise 90 degrees to scissor over comb in the nape area will help to blend these awkward hairlines to lie flat. Clipper over comb and scissor over comb techniques can be used. The angle at which you hold your comb is important and correct scissor hold is vital to the success of the haircut, to cut the hair as close as possible to the head without creating unwanted steps. Practice makes perfect when becoming competent in scissor and clipper over comb. Remember the outline shape, e.g. shorter at the nape gradually working up to the same length at the occipital bone.

There are many unisex haircuts that the cutting techniques can be used on, and then personalised for the end result (see Unit H26).

Drying the style

In order for the style to be created the hair must be dried in place. Remove the cutting cloth and remove all cut hair from your client. Take care when removing the cape not to drop cuttings onto your client. Use the neck brush in the nape area.

Replace the cutting cloth, and commence the dry. Apply any styling aids. A closely set bristle brush or heat-resistant comb may be used to guide the hair, together with a blow dryer with a nozzle to give control over the air flow. Commence the dry at the nape, taking care not to burn the scalp by allowing the air flow to rest in this area. Use the brush or comb to raise the roots, where required, to produce the shape and to tuck in the ends.

For a smooth result direct the airflow in the direction of the style. Adjust the position of the nozzle so that it does not touch your client's scalp or face during the drying.

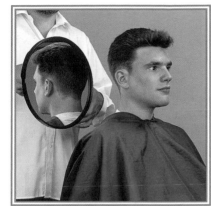

Once the dry is complete apply any hair products required and then dress the hair into position. A number of combs and brushes are available that will give textured effects to hair, if required. First brush the hair at 90 degrees to the desired direction and then firmly brush in the finished direction. Finger drying is a popular way to complete the haircut.

Finish by showing your client the finished result, having removed the gown and any protective clothes and by using the back mirror.

Figure 8.6 Using back mirror

Style variations

Partings

When a parting is used within the hairstyle it is usually to cut to this, leaving one side, the heavy side, longer than the other. The heavy side may require more thinning than the other. Many men's hairstyles have partings. These can be used in a variety of ways, e.g. to draw attention away from unwanted prominent facial features such as a large nose. Middle partings will create a more symmetrical look and also spread a mass of hair more evenly, which can make the hair more manageable. It is often best to use the natural partings as the hair tends to fall into the natural growth, especially if the hair is longer on the top.

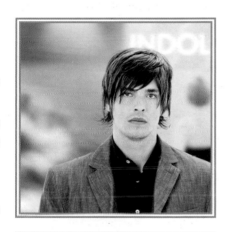

You need to assess the facial shape and agree a hairstyle that is complimentary to the facial shape and decide on an asymmetrical or symmetrical hair shape to balance the client's head and personal features.

Figure 8.7 Tapered fringe

Fringes

Fringes will normally be lined out by cutting on the forehead. Additional length may be required if the fringe is to cover a hairline that is receding. Fringes can be round, square, heavy, blunt or tapered. It is quite fashionable to spike up fringes that have been texturised to accentuate the client's profile. Fringes are normally tapered to give a softer line. However, if your client has a widow's peak or cow's lick you may need to leave the hair heavier as the hairline makes it difficult for the hair to sit flat and even. Remember it is usually better to go with the natural fall.

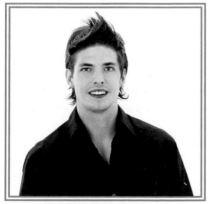

Off-face styles

Hair often dresses more easily back off the face if left a little longer than the rest of the hair. These can be in a smooth style or spiked away from the face, they can brush straight back or slightly to one side.

Figure 8.8 Spiked up fringe

Over-ear hairstyles

When cutting hair that will lie over the ear, allowance must be made for the hair to lie out over the ear and yet lie level with the rest of the hair. Often hair must be shaped around the ear or left substantially longer in order not to 'stick out' over the ear.

Added hairpieces

When cutting hair to fit with a hairpiece, that hair may require additional thinning so that it blends with the lengths of the added hair. Take care not to cut the added hair at the same time as the client's natural hair. Once complete ensure that the two do blend together.

Areas of hair loss

Often an additional length of hair must be left to allow an even line to be achieved over an area of hair loss. Discuss the requirements with your client before commencing the cut. Remember tact must be used at all times as hair loss can, for some, cause considerable mental anguish.

Review Questions

1 How should the electric clipper be used to outline the hair shape?

2 In what position should the hydraulic chair be when the client is invited to sit?

3 How should the client be protected before cutting the hair?

4 What is the largest size clipper grader available?

5 What should you do with your tools and equipment after each haircut?

6 Why do you need to be aware of growth patterns and the head shape when cutting hair?

7 Why is the scissor over comb used in preference to holding the hair with the fingers?

8 Should hair be wet or dry when using electric hair clippers?

9 What is the essential feature of a graduated neckline?

10 Is the razor used on wet or dry hair?

Additional information

Useful websites

Website Addresses	Content
www.habia.org.uk	Hairdressing and Beauty Industry Authority. Downloads available including references to other websites
www.bbc.safety.co.uk	Free advice on diseases in hairdressing
www.lookfantastic.com	Professional hairdressing products and advice
www.laurandp.co.uk	Educational publications for development of professional hairdressing
www.scott999.fsnet.co.uk	Hairdressing product information

The evidence from the activities below will cover the Underpinning Knowledge for the Technical Certificate for Advanced Modern Apprenticeships. You will need to take the external test and carry out the practical activities (see City and Guilds Diploma Hairdressing 6915/6913).

ACTIVITY

Outcome 1

Produce evidence for your portfolio on the following:

- Describe the correct use of cutting equipment.
- Explain how to maintain cutting equipment.
- Describe the effects created by different cutting techniques.
- State what factors need to be considered when cutting hair.
- Explain the safety considerations that must be taken into account when cutting hair.
- Describe the range of traditional looks for men, male teenagers and boys.
- State the importance of applying tension to the hair when cutting.
- Explain how to make sure the sideburns are cut level.
- State the importance of considering sideburns, outlines and neckline shapes and cutting the natural hairline when cutting men's hair.
- State the factors that need to be considered when cutting wet or dry hair.
- Explain how to dispose of sharps safely.
- Explain how to check and look after electrical equipment for safe use.

Outcome 2

Produce evidence for your portfolio on the following:

- Describe the correct use of cutting equipment.
- Explain how to maintain cutting equipment.
- Describe the effects created by different cutting techniques.
- State what factors need to be considered when cutting hair.
- Explain the safety considerations that must be taken into account when cutting hair.
- Describe the range of current fashion looks for men, male teenagers and boys.
- State the importance of applying tension to the hair when cutting.
- Explain how to make sure the sideburns are cut level.
- State the importance of considering sideburns, outlines and neckline shapes and cutting the natural hairline when cutting men's hair.
- State the factors that need to be considered when cutting wet or dry hair.
- Explain how to dispose of sharps safely.
- Explain how to check and look after electrical equipment for safe use.

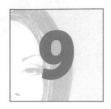

9 UNIT H22 DESIGN AND CREATE PATTERNS IN HAIR

1 Maintain effective and safe methods of working when creating designs in hair

2 Plan and agree hair pattern designs with your client

3 Create patterns in hair

Please read Units G1, H9, H21, and H30. Please follow the health and safety guidelines used within these units.

CHAPTER CONTENTS

- Designs
- Activity

Introduction

This unit relates to creating hair patterns that can be undertaken in a variety of ways – clippering, shaving, colouring and cutting. The most commonly used are clippering techniques, which are designed. The client consultation is extremely important as once these shapes have been created they are very difficult to change. Hair types and textures will give the design a personal finish, e.g. Afro-Caribbean hair looks extremely effective as the shape is very defined due to the hair structure.

Designs

The best way to create your design is to cut out a template or freehand draw the shape onto the client's hair. The hair is removed by using the clipper around and inside the shape, being careful not to cut into the design. Clippers, with no graders, are needed to remove the hair completely from the scalp. Coloured chalks or templates to mark out the design will be needed. Measuring and balancing the design are important.

You can use any type of design from pictures to lettering, etc. Flags, logos, names, pictures, animals, flowers, and symbols work well. Once you have made a template for a more complex design you can then start cutting it out. The hair that is left forms the design and needs to be short. A steady hand is needed. The hair should be moistened with water and the skin held taut. The hair is removed by shaving in the direction of the hairgrowth.

On Afro-Caribbean hair sometimes the hairlines are shaved or clippered giving a much stronger hairline e.g. square, pointed, to reflect a strong image. Once the hair has been removed you need to make sure the skin is not sore or does not bleed. Use talcum powder to soothe the skin. If the scalp is not normally shaved or clippered it can become sensitive and irritated. Be careful not to cut into the curve where the ear joins the scalp.

Once you have the design and you want to make it stand out, colour the hair using temporary, semi or permanent colours providing the necessary skin tests have been carried out (see Unit G9 for more details). This can make your hairstyle look totally different. In fact, if you did not want to shave the hair you could use the templates for colouring. Be careful to use your stencils carefully so as not to colour the whole area with one colour if you need several colours. Each colour will need its own template. The hair needs to be short for the best effect.

You may wish to leave some hair long, in which case you could undercut the hair then put a design in the short hair. You may want to shave or clipper a parting to strengthen the look, with the eybrow partially shaved to match. What ever you decide make sure the client is old enough to give consent otherwise get consent from the parent or guardian.

ACTIVITY

- Research design patterns for a number of looks.
- Make up a portfolio of these designs.
- Practise making a range of templates for hair designs and put them in your portfolios.
- Look at tattoo patterns and trace a design of your own.

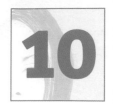

10 UNIT H34 PROVIDE FACE MASSAGING SERVICES

1 Maintain effective and safe methods of working when providing face massage services
2 Prepare the skin for massage services
3 Carry out face massage services

CHAPTER CONTENTS

- *Main Muscles*
- *Nerves*
- *Blood Supply*
- *Lymphatic System*
- *Contraindications of the Skin*
- *Preparing for Facial Massage*
- *Client Preparation*
- *The Massage*
- *Massage Movements*
- *Using the Vibro-Massager on the Face*
- *Further Study*
- *Review Questions*
- *Additional Information*
- *Activity*

Introduction

Many men and women enjoy the relaxing effects of a face massage or facial. In the barbers' shop this formed part of the shaving service but demand decreased as men started to shave at home more. However, the service seems to be showing signs of demand and a renewed interest within the salon. Facial massage may be used to improve muscle tone and relax your client. This service may be given to the client independently of any other service or following a wet shave.

A good facial routine is needed and preparation prior to the massage is vital to the success of this service. The consultation needs to be thorough to check for any contraindications and to reduce the risk of cross infection. Before you start your routine you must ensure you understand the basic anatomy of the face and neck and the effects that the massage has on its structures and systems.

It is important that you know the position of the muscles and how they act throughout the massage routine. The positions of the muscles are important and the movements should be performed along the muscle and towards its

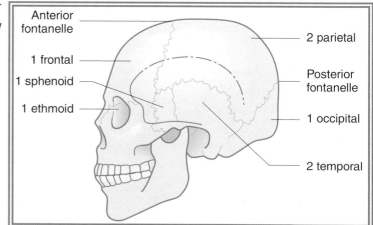

Figure 10.1 Bones of the cranium

origin. An understanding of the bones, nerves, blood supply and lymphatic system must also be understood, as this will affect your choice of technique and the speed and depth of the pressure applied.

- Bones of the face: maxillae, mandible, malar and nasal.
- Bones of the cranium: frontal, sphenoid and temporal.

As you massage the face you will feel the shapes of bones beneath your fingers. Sometimes there is little tissue between the bones and the surface of the skin. You must take care in these areas to choose the right massage technique to avoid discomfort to the client.

The muscles are an essential part of the face that allow you to eat and speak and to produce facial expressions. They are interlinked with each other and with the bones. One end of the mouth is attached to a static bone by a strong tendon, called the muscle's origin. The other end is attached to a moveable bone, to another muscle or to the skin, which is called the muscle's intersection.

Massage movements are made towards the origin and away from the point of insertion. Discomfort can be caused to your client if you massage the wrong way.

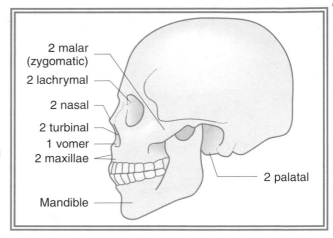

Figure 10.2 Bones of the face

Main muscles

- Occipital frontalis – covers the top of the cranium. It enables you to lift the eyebrows.
- Orbicularis oculi – surrounds the eye and helps to form the eyelids and allows the eyelid to close.
- Orbicularis oris – surrounds the mouth. It allows you to close the mouth and speak.
- Temporalis – connects to the temporal bone and with the malar and mandible bones. This helps you to close your mouth and chew.
- Masseter – lies between the mandible and malar bone and helps to close the jaw.
- Zygomaticus – lies between the malar bones and corners of the mouth and allows the lip to move outwards.

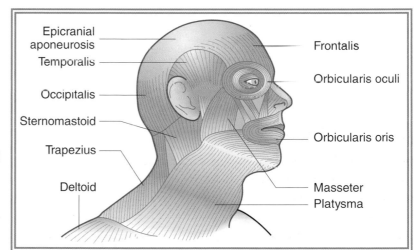

Figure 10.3 Muscles of the head and face

- Steromastoid – runs behind the ears to the temporal bones. It helps to rotate the head and bow.
- Platysma – muscle within the front of the neck that allows you to wrinkle the skin and lower the corners of the mouth.

Nerves

Nerves carry messages to the skin, muscles, teeth, nose and the mouth. The 5th cranial nerve (trigeminal) and 7th cranial nerve (facial nerve) are the main nerves associated with the face. Gentle massage may be applied to these areas depending on the technique used, which are smooth or stimulated.

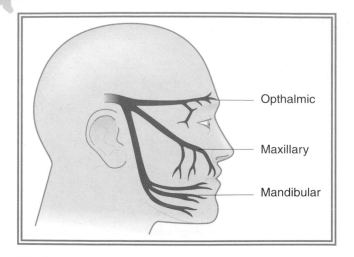

Figure 10.4 The 5th cranial (trigeminal) nerve

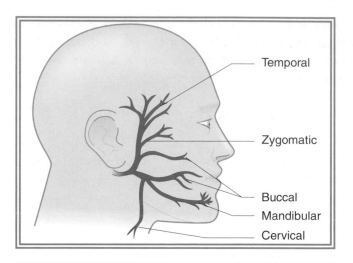

Figure 10.5 The 7th cranial (facial) nerve

Blood supply

The heart pumps oxygenated blood around through the arteries. This nourishes all the areas of the body. The main blood supply to the face and head is through the carotid arteries, which then divide into smaller arteries (arterioles) and then into capillaries. The capillaries join to venules then veins, which then carry the blood back to the heart. The main veins that run down the side of the neck from the head and face and are called jugular veins.

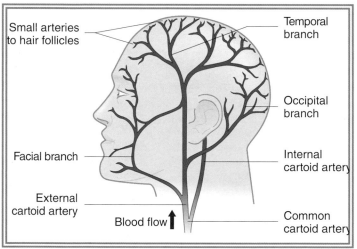

Figure 10.6 Blood supply to the head

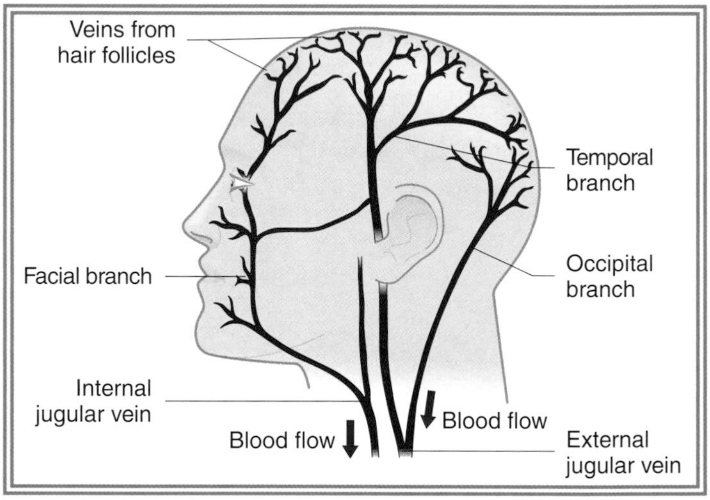

Figure 10.7 Blood vessels from the head

The heart pumps the oxygen-depleted blood to the lungs where the oxygen is replaced and returns to the heart. The process then starts all over again.

Lymphatic system

The main function of the lymphatic system is to remove bacteria, foreign matter and excess fluids from the tissues. This is particularly important as it helps to prevent infection. Lymph is a pale yellow fluid, which travels away from the tissue towards the heart.

The lymphatic system is made up of a network of lymph vessels, lymph nodes and lymph glands, which closely follow the veins throughout the body. The lymphatic system can be stimulated through massage and can help to promote the flow of lymph to the nodes. This helps to remove waste products and toxins from the facial tissue.

Contraindications of the skin

If you discover any of the indications below, do not proceed with the massage but refer your client to the doctor using tact and diplomacy. Infections can spread easily. There is more information in Unit G9.

- Broken skin or bleeding.
- Inflammation, swelling and bruising.
- Eye disorders such as conjunctivitis.
- Skin disorders such as impetigo.
- Acne, swelling, skin disorders.

Preparing for facial massage

You will require:

- a clean gown or cape
- clean towels
- suitable massage lotion for-
  - ▶ dry skin – a moisturising cream
  - ▶ greasy skin – a 'roll out' cream
  - ▶ normal skin – a massage cream
- mild astringent lotion
- fine talc
- vibro massager with sponge and/or bell applicator
- supply of steam towels
- supply of cold towels
- clean spatula
- tissue.

Client preparation

Ensure that your hands are clean and that any open sores are covered with a waterproof dressing. When offering this service to your client for the first time, take time to explain the process, giving them, in understandable terms, an overview of the massage, and the benefits that they will obtain, the time it will take and if the client is unaware, the costs. Seat your client on the hydraulic chair and discuss their skin type. Check whether the skin is dry, greasy, normal or combination. This will determine the type of massage lotion you will use. Check for contraindications and gown your client in the same manner as for a wet shave.

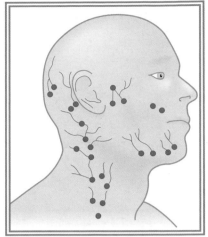

Figure 10.8 The lymph nodes

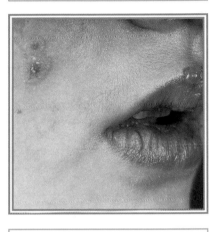

Figure 10.9 Boil

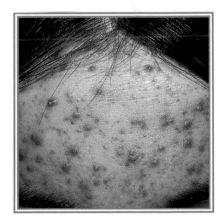

Figure 10.10 Acbe vvlgaris

Procedure

Directions:

1 Recline the chair and guide your client into position. Adjust the height of the chair, to enable you to reach over to your client's face while standing behind the chair and without your body resting on theirs.

2 Place a clean tissue over the headrest of the chair, to prevent the spread of infection from one head to another.

3 Gown your client in the same manner as for a wet shave. If your client's hair falls forward onto the forehead, this should be held back and protected from the massage cream by using a head band or a clean towel wrapped around the head.

4 Apply a hot steam towel to the client's face. This will help to relax your client, open the pores, and cleanse the skin. Remove this before it cools and apply massage cream to the face, spotting it over the areas to be massaged.

   The massage cream will lubricate the surface of the skin, allowing the hands and other massage tools to move smoothly, causing no discomfort to your client. These creams contain additives, which will be beneficial to the skin.

5 Use a clean spatula to remove the massage cream from its container. This will help to prevent cross infection. Place the cream on the back of your hand. Using the fingers from your other hand gently smooth the cream over the area to be massaged and then apply a further steam towel. This will help in the penetration of the skin's surface by the massage cream as well as relaxing your client.

6 Remove the hot towel before it cools, taking care not to wipe the cream from the face.

Remember: Remove massage cream from the tub using a clean spatula, placing the cream onto the back of your hand. This will help to prevent cross infection caused by passing skin disorders from the client's skin into the product within the tub.

Remember: Your face will be in very close proximity to that of your client; always ensure that your hair does not fall onto their face, that your breath is clear of unpleasant odours, including those from cigarettes and strong flavoured food.

If necessary apply additional massage cream to the face and then, standing at the back of your client, commence the facial massage.

Remember: The process of facial massage should be one that relaxes your client; all massage movements should follow a smooth, rhythmic, uninterrupted pattern. A hand should remain in contact with your client's face at all times during the actual massage process.

The massage

There are three massage movements that are used during the process of facial massage. These are:

- Effleurage – a light continuous stroking movement applied with either the fingers or the palm of the hand in a slow rhythmic manner. No pressure is used. The palms work over large surfaces (see Figure 10.11), while the cushions of the fingertips work over small surfaces (around the eyes) (see Figure 10.12). This has a soothing, relaxing effect.

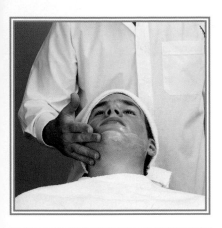

Figure 10.11 Effleurage massage, large areas

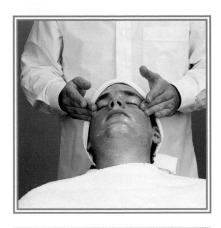

Figure 10.12 Effleurage massage, small areas

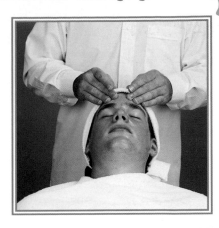

Figure 10.13 Petrissage massage

- Petrissage – a kneading movement of the skin and underlying flesh between your fingers and the palm of the hand. As you lift the tissues from their underlying structures, squeeze, roll or pinch with a light, firm pressure (see Figure 10.13). This movement invigorates the part being treated.

- Tapotement or percussion – consists of tapping, slapping and hacking movements (see Figure 10.14). This form of massage is most stimulating. It should be applied with care, particularly over areas where there is little muscle tissue.

The frequency of facial massage depends upon the condition of the skin, the age of your client and the condition to be treated (if applicable). As a general rule, normal skin can be kept in excellent condition with a weekly massage, accompanied by proper home care.

Massage movements

Standing at the back of the hydraulic chair place the fingers of your hands at each of the client's temples. Movements should be rhythmic and soothing, not jerky and sharp.

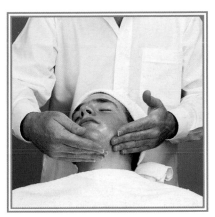

Figure 10.14 Tapotement massage

Directions:

1 *Massage across the forehead in small circular movements, first with one hand from left to right and then with the other hand from right to left. The hands should always return to the resting point at the temples.*

2 *Massage across the forehead using a zig-zag up and down movement, first from left to right and then from right to left.*

3 *Place the first two fingers of your left hand over to the right hand side of the tip of the nose and with the pads of the finger using only slight pressure draw this upward to the forehead and across the bridge of the nose to the forehead. As one hand almost finishes the*

movement the other hand should start on the other side. Avoid too much pressure on the tip of the nose as the cartilage can easily be damaged.

4 *In a co-ordinated manner, simultaneously slide the first two fingers of each hand from the bridge of the nose, down the sides of the nose,*

Contraindications: Massage should never be given when there is evidence of muscular swelling, cuts, abrasions or contagious disorders present.

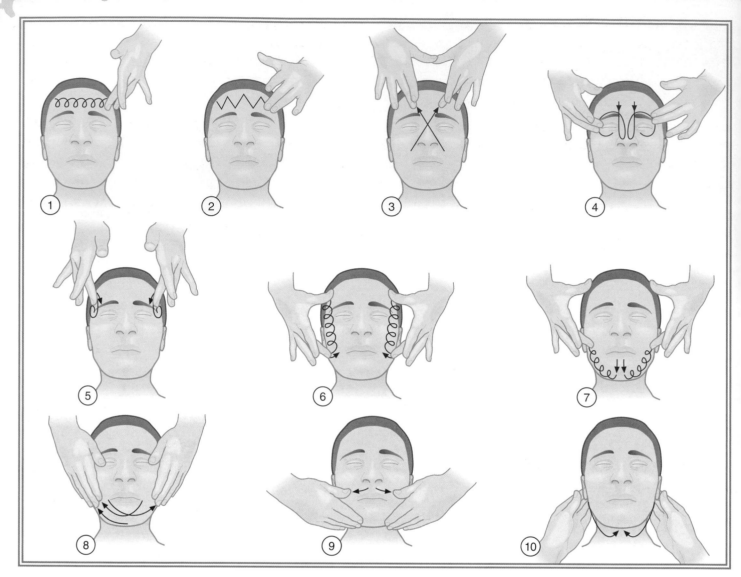

Figure 10.15 Face massage movements

in a circular action back up the same side, near the ridge and then around the eye.

5 Return the hands to the temples, and simultaneously massage the temples, at each side, in small circular movements.

6 Simultaneously slide the fingers at both sides down to the corner of the jaw and then using circular movements rotate them back up to the temples.

7 Slide the fingers to the centre of the chin, and simultaneously using circular movements massage above the jawbone back to the corner of the jaw.

8 Cupping the hand, either side at a time, draw the palm and fingers from the corner of the mouth, across the chin to the corner of the jaw,

the second finger running in line with the jaw bone and drawing up under the chin. Repeat this on either side.

9 Draw the thumbs across the area above the top lip, from the centre outwards to each side.

10 Reaching across your client, cup the hand around the neck and draw your hand from just behind the ear, across the front and upwards across the underside of the centre chin.

Remember: Should your client experience discomfort during the massage it should be terminated.

Each movement should be carried out approximately five times; avoid too much pressure on the skin. Remember the purpose is to relax, therefore carry this out in a relaxing style. Once the massage is completed, apply a hot steam towel to the face. This will help with the removal of any excess massage cream or oil. Before it is cool, remove the towel and, having folded it lengthways use it to wipe the cream from the face. Ensure removal from the areas around the hairline, the nose and ears.

A cold towel may then be applied; this will help to close the pores of the skin, therefore leaving it less exposed to infection. The cold towels may be prepared in a similar method to the hot steam towel, by folding, moistening and rolling the towel, and then placing in a cool cabinet. Following its removal a mild astringent, for example rose water or witch hazel, may be applied using the palms of your hands. This will serve further to close the pores.

Using clean tissue, blot the skin of the face dry and then apply a small quantity of fine talc to soothe and remove shine from the skin. Apply the talc from the palms of your hands or from a talc puffer while the client's nose and eyes are protected by your cupped hand.

Finally, check that all excess product is removed from your client's skin. Remove the protective towels from your client and then raise the back of the chair, slowly. Remove the cape and give your client a tissue to wipe his face, should he wish. Give your client the opportunity to assess the effect of the treatment just completed.

> *Remember: Lower the hydraulic chair, to its lowest position, before allowing your client to step off.*

Clean up, placing waste in a covered bin and used linen in the laundry basket. Return containers to the storage area and clean all equipment.

Using the vibro-massager on the face

The vibro-massager may be used, with care, to give facial massage. This should never be used if there is the presence of any contraindications to the service including, muscular swelling, open cuts or sores or the presence of any contagious disorders.

The bell shaped vibro applicator is use for this process.

Prepare the client and the face as for facial massage already described. Firmly attach the bell shape applicator to the

> *Remember: Always check the vibro massager and its flex for damage before use. Only use with dry hands.*

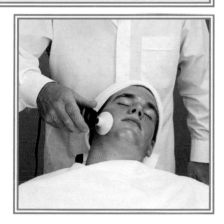

Figure 10.16 Vibro massager in use

massager. Due to the delicate nature of the facial skin, the vibro massager must be used gently on the skin. Avoid pressure on areas where the jaw bone, etc, is prominent.

Directions:

1 *Use circular movements across the upper jaw area.*

2 *Draw the vibro across the neck in sweeping motions either side of the windpipe.*

3 *Support the side of the nose with the free hand and gently draw the vibro along the side of the nose from the tip up towards the forehead. Take care that the applicator does not jar on any prominent bone or cartilage.*

4 *Place the applicator on the back of your free hand and massage the muscle around the eyes using the fingers of this hand.*

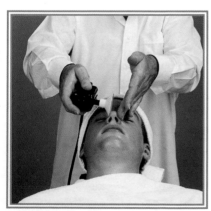

Figure 10.17 Vibro massager in use on side of nose

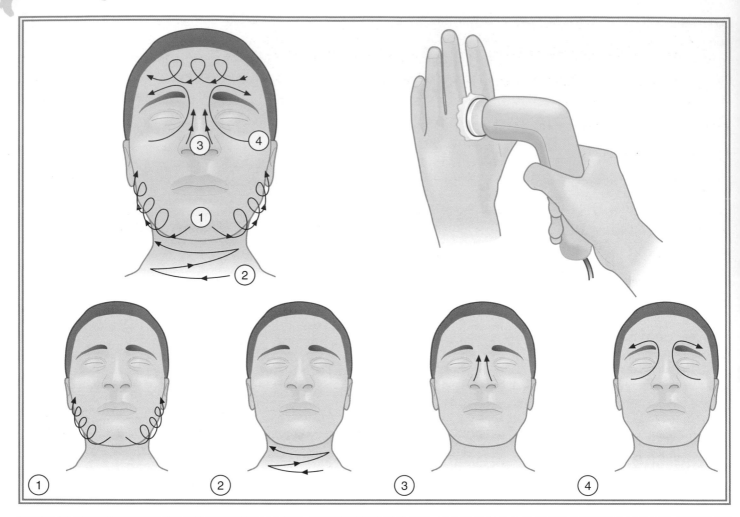

Figure 10.18 Vibro-massager movements

Finish and tidy away material as described previously. Remember to wipe the casing of the vibro massager and to wash, dry and sterilise the applicator (bell shaped attachment).

Further study

- To obtain best results from facial massage, you must have a thorough knowledge of all the structures involved: muscles, nerves and blood vessels.

- Every muscle and nerve has a motor point. In order to obtain the maximum benefit from a facial massage you must consider the motor nerve points that affect the underlying muscles of the face and neck.

- Local bye-laws may regulate the offering of barbering skills; find out from your local area what these bye-laws require.

Review Questions

1   State two contraindications to carrying out a face massage.

2   What steps should be taken should your client's skin become sensitive?

3   Suggest two facial massage movements.

4   What benefit is gained by the use of steam towels?

5   What is the purpose of carrying out a facial massage?

6   What benefits, for your client, are achieved by facial massage?

7   What is the purpose of using cold towels following a facial massage?

8   When should a facial massage be carried out?

Additional information

Useful websites

Website Addresses	Content
www.habia.org.uk	Hairdressing and Beauty Industry Authority. Downloads available including references to other websites
www.bbc-safety.co.uk	Free advice on diseases in hairdressing
www.trichologists.org.uk	Institute of Trichologists
www.lookfantastic.com	Professional hairdressing products and advice
www.laurandp.co.uk	Educational publications for development of professional hairdressing
www.scott999.fsnet.co.uk	Hairdressing product information

The evidence from the activities below will cover the Underpinning Knowledge for the Technical Certificate for Advanced Modern Apprenticeships. You will need to take the external test and carry out the practical activities (see City and Guilds Diploma Hairdressing 6913).

ACTIVITY

Produce evidence for your portfolio on the following:

Outcome 1

- *Explain how to maintain and check safety of electrical massage equipment.*
- *Describe the effects and the benefits created by different massage techniques on the client, their skin and its underlying structures and state how to use them.*
- *State what factors need to be considered when providing massage services.*
- *Describe the safety considerations that must be taken into account when providing massage services.*
- *List the range of finishing products available and state the effects that they have on the skin.*
- *List the problems that may occur during massage services and state how to resolve them.*
- *State the importance of using personal protective equipment when providing face massage and after shaving services.*
- *State the suitability of different massage techniques for different areas of the face.*
- *State the reasons for and the effects of using hot and cool towels.*
- *State when massage services should not be carried out.*
- *List the methods of sterilisation and sanitation available and state which are suitable for use in the barbers' shop.*
- *State the importance of avoiding cross infection and infestations.*

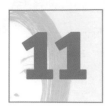

11 UNIT H24 DEVELOP AND ENHANCE YOUR CREATIVE SKILLS

1 Plan and design a range of images

2 Produce a range of creative images

3 Evaluate your results against the design plan objectives

CHAPTER CONTENTS

- *Developing Awareness of Creative Images*
- *Developing Storyboards*
- *Introducing Themes and Presenting Creative Images*
- *Evaluating your Design*
- *Additional Information*
- *Activity*

Developing awareness of creative images

To develop your skills you need to look at hair as a medium that can be moulded and shaped to create fashion, period, avant-garde and classic looks.

Ask yourself:

- How do you go about this to make your ideas become reality?
- How do you make the ideas become visually acceptable?
- Who says what is fashion and what is avant-garde?
- Why do some trends take off and others do not?

There are many answers and arguments to these questions but first of all you need to appreciate what is around you and interpret what art forms interest you and why. There are designs that will visually and personally affect you at any moment. Each person is different and they perceive things in a different way. That is what makes art and design so interesting and gives us new and exciting ideas.

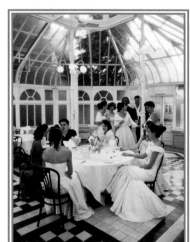

Figure 11.1

How do you start to create a collection of creative images for your audience to interpret? You could start by looking at what influences you, e.g. television, celebrities, music, clothes, textures, furniture, the environment. What colours do you like, what materials do you like to feel, what artists appeal to you, what types of designs do you like, and what are we designing these images for?

Developing storyboards

Build a storyboard and collect as much information and samples as you can. Try to think of what is new and how that can be reflected in your design. Draw and research some images. Look in art galleries, look at plays and musicals. Look in museums and in historical reference books.

Decide on a theme/subject, e.g. black and white, tribal, Andy Warhol, Van Gogh, Mary Quant, flowers, metals, Clarice Cliff, 1930s, something that inspires you. Once you have chosen a theme/subject, collect ideas that relate so you can build a storyboard.

Black and white

1. Carry out a brainstorming session with a group of people to collect all their ideas. Ask them to write down anything that springs to mind relating to black and white. What first springs to my mind is 1960s, Mary Quant, Scottie dogs, draughts, black and white photographs, mock Tudor houses. Put this list on a large pin board.

2. Collect images that relate to black and white from the media, etc. Pin these to your notice board.

3. Choose fabrics that relate to these ideas and pin them to the notice board.

4. Choose shapes and pin these to the notice board.

5. Stand the board up where you can see it each day.

6. Subconsciously you will be thinking about black and white. Collect any additional information that you think is relevant.

7. Now interpret this by relating your thoughts and ideas through to your hairstyles.

8. You need to design a classic look linked to black and white and incorporate this in your storyboard. Mary Quant used to wear a classic one-length bob, big round eyes and a black and white shift dress. You could work on an updated version or replicate the Mary Quant look.

9. You now need to link to a fashionable updated version of Mary Quant, e.g. strong lines, black hair, white highlighted fringe to strengthen the shape, etc.

10. You now need to link to avant-garde Mary Quant, e.g. strengthen the bob, reverse the colours – white hair black fringe – over the top and exaggerated makeup, very strong hair cut at geometrical disconnected lengths to exaggerate the shapes, etc.

11. Make sure you photograph the different stages of your work.

12. Look at your photographs and see what needs to be improved in your work.

13. Collect all the evidence listed in the points above for assessment.

Introducing themes and presenting creative images

Present your collection of black and white photographs and label the main points of the theme, i.e. Mary Quant, geometrics, classic, fashion, avant-garde.

Once you have got the ideas onto your storyboard you need to work on your models to practise the hairstyles. You may need to cut and colour the hair. You may also need to use postiche, added hair, etc. You will need to organise what you want your models to wear. Look in charity shops, jumble sales and car boot sales. You will be surprised what you might find useful and relatively inexpensive. Once you are happy with the results, organise a presentation to show your models.

If you feel really brave, organise a fashion show. Black and white is just a simple idea that can look really effective. Look at the Mohican and how that trend has developed and where it originally came from. You need to spend some time researching, preparing and organising your collection. This unit can be great fun, especially if you want to expand your creative ability.

You may be thinking of designing these images for photographic shoots for your own salon, the media, theatre, television, etc.

Evaluating your design

Evaluate evidence through discussion, questionnaires and feedback. Compare people's perceptions and impressions against your original objectives. Ask yourself, did people perceive the theme correctly, could they detect the origins of the theme, was the message understood, and was it aesthetically pleasing. Use the findings from evaluation to inform your future actions and design decisions.

Additional information

Useful websites

Website Addresses	Content
www.habia.org.uk	Hairdressing and Beauty Industry Authority. Downloads available including references to other websites
www.bbc-safety.co.uk	Free advice on diseases in hairdressing
www.keyskillssupport.net	Key skills information and downloads
www.lookfantastic.com	Professional hairdressing products and advice
www.vidalsassoon.com.	Range of hairdressing products and education
www.trevorsorbie.com	Range of hairdressing products, hairstyles and education
www.nexus.com	Range of hairdressing products and hairstyles
www.tigi.co.uk	Range of hairdressing products
www.schwarzkopf.com	Range of hairdressing products

Magazines and journals

- *Hairdressers Journal*
- *Creative Head*
- *Estetica/Cutting Edge*
- *Black Beauty and Hair*

ACTIVITY

Outcome for Key Skills Communication Level 2 and H23 NVQ 3 Hairdressing

- *Prepare a short talk on designing your creative image using props, e.g. your storyboard and the process you went through.*
- *Carry out a discussion on your chosen theme and invite feedback. Record useful points.*
- *Design a questionnaire for your group to complete.*
- *Present your collection.*
- *If you are studying a Modern Apprenticeship or Communication Key Skills Level 2 then get your tutor to assess you on the points above.*

UNIT H25 STYLE AND DRESS HAIR TO CREATE A VARIETY OF LOOKS

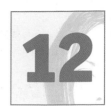

1 Maintain effective and safe methods of working when styling hair

2 Style and dress hair creatively

CHAPTER CONTENTS

- Setting Principles
- The Styling Process
- Gowning Your Client
- Choice of Styling Technique
- Styling Aids
- Styling Tools
- Blow Drying

- Finger Drying
- Scrunch Drying
- Natural Drying
- Setting Hair
- Heated Appliances
- Review Questions
- Activity

Introduction

The client wishes to leave the hair stylist looking their best. Fulfilling this wish ensures client satisfaction and helps to establish good customer relations. The way that the client looks when they leave the hair stylist indicates, both to the client and to potential clients, the professional ability and character of the hair stylist. The finished hairstyle becomes an advertisement for the stylist's work and the salon's standard of hairdressing.

The choice of drying and dressing technique used will depend upon the finished outcome required (this will be agreed with the client by consultation, see Unit G9), the hair type being dressed and the preferences of the client. This selection and choice of hairstyle and technique will be made from advice given to and negotiation with your client during consultation, which would normally take place before the hairdressing process begins and may be reviewed throughout the treatment.

As your client will become an advertisement of your hairdressing skills it is important that they are able to maintain their hair at its best between visits. Educate your client in how to maintain the style, particularly following the introduction of a new look to the client. Home use products, which complement the products used in your salon and will enable the style to be maintained, should be recommended and offered for sale. Always ensure that the client is aware of how to use these products correctly.

Setting principles

- Shampooing – this cleanses and wets the hair allowing it to be 'stretched' and formed into a new shape. Hydrogen and salt bonds within the cortex of the hair are temporarily broken down by the water, allowing the hair to be stretched.

Hair stretches more easily when wet, and shampooing the hair wets it more effectively than just damping with a trigger spray.

- Drying – during this stage the hair is stretched into a new shape and dried into that shape. The hydrogen and sulphur bonds in the hair reform and hold the hair in the shape in which it was dried.

- Reforming – when the hair is wetted again it returns to its natural shape and may be restyled again. Hair absorbs moisture from the atmosphere (it is hygroscopic) and therefore the hairstyle gradually falls, falling more rapidly in moist damp conditions (high humidity). Styling aids often place a coating on the hair to slow down this absorption of moisture, delaying elastic recoil, and therefore increasing the life of the style.

The styling process

Client consultation – establishing the required hairstyle (see Unit G9).

Gowning your client

The purpose of gowning your clients is to protect them and their clothing from damage or contamination during the hairdressing process. The exact method of gowning used will depend upon your salon's policy and the nature of the hairdressing processes you are about to carry out and may be varied during your client's visit to the salon.

When carrying out treatments where the hair is wet your client will require a gown to prevent moisture causing discomfort, or damage to clothing. However, when using styling irons gowning has different requirements, as there will not be any moisture present.

Gowning will normally follow the initial consultation with your client; this may depend upon your salon's policy. During your consultation it is useful to be aware of the style of clothing that they wear, as this can give you a feel for their fashion sense, which in turn can guide you in your style suggestions. Note, however, if your client has had damage to their clothing in the past while visiting the salon, they may not be wearing their usual clothes.

Clean gowning materials should be used to help prevent the spread of infectious disorders from one client to the next. Different salons' methods of gowning may vary; however, all will endeavour to ensure that the client's clothing is protected.

Choice of styling technique

Your choice of the techniques you will use to achieve the result discussed with your client will depend upon a number of factors. These include:

- Finished style required – some techniques are better suited to particular hairstyles.

- Hair texture – fine hair may require more support in the drying technique, whereas thick, strong, coarse hair will require less and will produce much of its own volume.

- Hair type – curly hair may require more tension when drying to control or reduce the natural curl. Strong hair growth patterns, for example, a 'double crown', may require more control in the drying process.

Styling aids

Styling aids have the following properties, they:

- help to make the hair more manageable during the drying process

- prolong the life of the hairstyle, by excluding atmospheric moisture

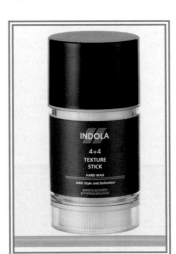

Figure 12.1 Hair wax

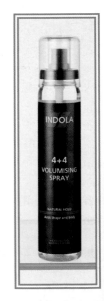

Figure 12.2 Volumising spray

● give the hair the necessary stiffness to enable the required hairstyle to be produced

● help to condition and moisturise the hair

● compensate for the damaging effect that heat can have on the hair.

Your choice of styling aids will be determined by the client's hair type, the required hairstyle, the features of the particular product, your personal preference and the salon's product range and use policy.

Blow-dry lotions are available in liquid form, as a single application phial and multi-application bottles, as well as aerosol and pump action. Liquids are applied by sprinkling onto the hair, spreading throughout using both your fingers and comb. Aerosols may be applied by directing the spray onto the hair, ensuring distribution by directing the spray throughout the head of hair and by combing. Take care: avoid applying too much of the product which will then run onto the client's neck, weigh down the hair and cause waste.

Mousse is a blow-dry lotion in foam form, making the product easier to apply and distribute by hand throughout all the hair or on specific areas of the hair. Apply a sphere of mousse the size of a golf ball by hand, distributing it throughout the hair using the fingers, followed by a wide-toothed comb. Take care when first applying the mousse as it can be inclined to roll off the hair.

Gel is a styling aid that has a heavier consistency than mousse or blow-dry lotions. Applied from the palms of your hands, it is distributed throughout the hair. The gel may also be applied to specific parts of the hair using the pads or tips of your fingers. Gel can be available in both a normal dry look when dry, and a wet look. The crisp finish left on the hair, if the gel is left to dry undisturbed, makes gel very suitable for sculptured/slick looks.

These products are often available for a variety of hair types and degrees of hold, normal and firm.

Curl activators and moisturisers are usually available as a pump action spray. Spray this onto curly hair to give a more controlled, defined curl. Direct the spray throughout the hair and distribute using a wide-toothed comb and the fingers. These products are particularly useful on hair that is dry, difficult to control and fragile.

Styling tools

Your choice of blow-dryer may depend upon your personal preference, what is available and the type of style to be produced. Hairdryers are available with a range of controls including differing air speeds and heat settings. For controlled drying a 'fishtail-style' nozzle can be fitted to many dryers to reduce the disruption to the hair caused by the air flow.

Select styling tools that will not be adversely affected by the levels of heat used in the drying process. Remember that many plastic and nylon-based tools will distort if exposed to heat for too long. The fine nylon bristles of brushes may soften or the teeth of plastic combs may bend. Vulcanite (hardened rubber) combs have a slightly higher heat resistance. Metal tools, such as aluminium combs, may be used when controlling short hair or producing waves of raised partings, but they can become very hot, and may burn the skin if they touch the client's scalp. Bone combs have a high resistance to heat.

There are a number of brushes designed specifically for use when blow drying, including 'vent' style brushes, which are designed to aid air flow and thus speed up hair drying, and radial brushes of a variety of diameters that enable you to dry the hair into curved or rounded shapes. Watch hairstylists, demonstrators and your instructors drying hair and the range of drying tools that they use. This may guide you in your choices.

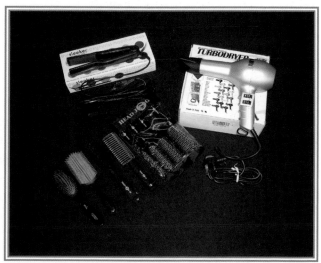

Figure 12.3 Styling tools

Blow drying

This technique is suitable for a wide range of hairstyles on a variety of hair types and hair lengths. The hairdryer is used together with a variety of tools, including hands, combs and brushes, the choice of which depends on the style required.

Best results will be achieved on hair that is freshly shampooed. Shampooing prepares the hair by cleansing it and enabling it to be stretched into a new shape. The hair can then be dried into this new shape, delaying elastic recoil, which it will retain until the hair is moistened again.

Following the shampoo, remove the excess moisture from the hair by towel drying. Remove any tangles from the hair using a wide-toothed comb, taking extra care not to cause discomfort to the client, or damage to the hair, by excessive tension on the hair. Fine porous hair is very easily damaged and broken while wet.

Apply appropriate styling aids to the hair, taking care not to allow the product to spill onto the client's face or neck, and comb the hair into the direction of the style. Manufacturers have a great range of products for styling the hair to give you the choice of look you are trying to achieve. It is great to have such a wide range of creative products that condition and style the hair. This allows you to combine your hairdressing techniques to give an extensive range of hairstyles. Apply products to the hair evenly and not to the scalp. Make sure you use products in a well-ventilated room and protect the client from any spray that could go into the eyes or on the skin (see Unit G1 relating to the use of products).

Take care to avoid overheating the hair, as excessive heat can damage the hair and cause your client discomfort. Avoid holding the air flow against the hair in one place for too long, as this may cause excessive heating and subsequent damage to the hair.

Having removed excess moisture start your blow dry at the lower parts of the hairstyle, those areas that will be on the underneath the style (see Figure 12.4). Make partings and take a section and secure with a clip. Work on the hair using the correct tool to give the amount of lift, curl and body that is desired. Place the brush in the direction that you want the hair to fall and hold the dryer about 10 cm away from the hair to avoid over drying or damaging the hair. If there is an area of the head or a part of the style that is likely to be particularly resistant to styling, this is often best dried first. Ensure that each mesh of hair is dried before moving on to the next, as meshes that are left damp will affect others that lie adjacent.

Perfect blow drying means working neatly. There are a number of brushes and tools to help you decide on finished look, i.e. radial large brushes for volume and shine. Using styling lotions will help to retain the blow dry by putting coatings on the hair to give texture and shine. For smooth results the air flow should be directed with the direction of the hair. When achieving lift and volume, hold up meshes of hair in turn and direct the dryer into the root area (see Figure 12.5).

Use the dressing mirror to check the shape and balance of the hair style being developed.

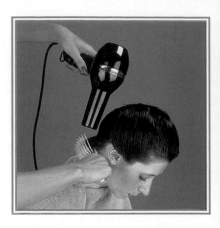

Figure 12.4 Blow drying at the nape

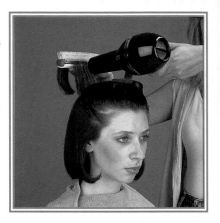

Figure 12.5 Blow drying to achieve root lift

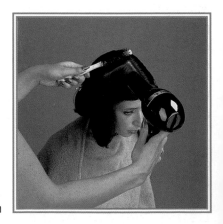

Figure 12.6 Blow drying with a radial brush

Using the radial brush

Using the radial brush will enable you to dry the hair into curls or waves. Your choice of brush will depend upon a number of factors:

- The strength of curl achieved will depend on the radius of the brush that you use: the larger the radius, the softer the curl; the smaller the radius the tighter the curl. Curl strength may also depend on the amount of hair wrapped around the hairbrush when drying.

- The length of hair may determine the size of brush, as the hair will need to be long enough to be wrapped around the brush.

- Differing types of bristle material have differing characteristics. Fine, closely set bristle tends to grip the hair; widely spaced bristle may control the hair more easily and remove tangles.

- Your choice will often be personal choice. If in doubt, check with your supervisor.

Use the radial brush as follows:

Using the fingers, section off a mesh of hair and place it on the brush. Rotate the brush to smooth the ends of the hair into the direction of movement. Wind the hair around the brush and direct the air flow from the hairdryer in the direction in which the hair is lying (see Figure 12.6). Directing the air flow against the direction of the hair will produce a messy result as the shorter hairs within the mesh will be dried without control and may produce a fuzzy appearance in the style.

To avoid damage to the hair by excessive heat do not direct the airflow at one place all the time. Keep the airflow moving over the hair. Rotate the brush to ensure that the hair is dried into a smooth finish around it. When working with long or very thick hair, drying can be more effective if you dry the ends of the hair first, gradually winding the hair around the brush and drying it progressively, working towards the root area. Take care when drying very long hair that the brush does not become entangled in it.

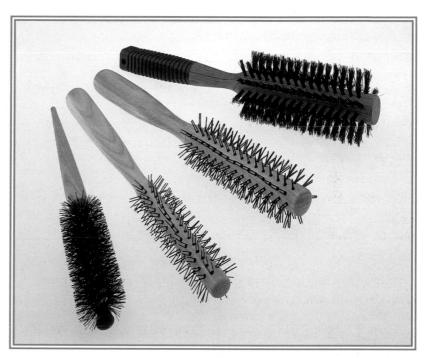

Figure 12.7 Radial brushes

When drying fine hair (which drops the curl easily) or hair that is resistant to curl, leaving the brush as the hair cools will enhance curl retention. Using blasts of cool air from the hairdryer can speed this process.

If you wish to achieve lift at the roots, lift the mesh away from the head. The higher the mesh is lifted (over directed) the greater the lift achieved with the particular brush. Larger diameter brushes will produce more root lift. Flatter results will be produced by using root drag or incorporating the use both of the radial and flat brush on the hair.

Using the flat brush

Using the flat brush will enable you to produce smooth, straight hair styles. There are two main styles of flat brush:

- Brushes with closely set, fine bristles can be very useful when styling very short hair that may not be long enough to lie easily on the brush.

- Brushes with widely spaced, thick bristles, are ideal when styling smooth straight styles where the hair length is sufficient to lie on the brush.

Generally the differences between brushes of these categories lie in their size, the number of rows of bristles and the style of base. Your choice should be the one that is the most comfortable for you to use. The styles of base available are rubber-cushioned back, solid back or vented back. The rubber-cushioned back allows the bristles to move slightly and therefore flex with the hair. Both this and the solid back give smoother results on straight hairstyles. The vented back aids drying of the hair.

Using your fingers, take small meshes of hair and lay them in the bristle of the brush. With the air flow of the hairdryer directed onto the mesh of hair and in the direction of the hair, draw the brush from the roots to the points of the hair. You will produce a smooth, straight result in this manner. When straightening wavy hair, slight tension must be maintained on the hair. If a slight movement is required, for example to turn the ends of a bobbed hairstyle either out or under, then roll the brush in the appropriate direction and direct the air flow onto the corner of the brush.

You may use either a brush or comb to control wet hair while blow drying:

● use a brush on long hair

● use a comb on short hair.

Shape the hair and direct the airflow into the trough of the wave.

Finger drying

This technique is best suited to hair that falls into style easily, has some natural volume and movement, and where an informal look is required. Your hands become the tools that guide the hair into position during the drying process. In many cases body heat from your hands aids the drying of the hair. Drying is often aided by the use of the hair dryer. Your fingers will draw the hair into place either in a 'claw-like' fashion, the fingers taking on the role of a wide-toothed comb or brush, or will mould the hair by wrapping it around the fingers to produce movement in the hair.

Lift and volume at the roots is achieved by rotary movements of the hair at the root, movement using finger pads or the palm of your hand and lifting the hair away from the scalp. Your client's head is normally maintained in an upright position except when producing volume in medium-length and long hair, when the head may be inclined downwards and then brought upright when the root area is dry.

Scrunch drying

This technique is used when a full curly style is required, usually on medium or long hair lengths. Compress the wet hair, into its curled shape in the hand and direct the air flow onto the palm of the hand, opening the hand to allow the access of the warm air and then closing to scrunch. Continue to scrunch the hair as it cools after the heat has been removed. This will improve retention of movement.

When dressing a finished hairstyle you may use this scrunching technique to encourage movement in the hair. Place a small amount of styling aid, mousse, gel or wax onto the palms of your hands and then, without added heat, scrunch the hair.

Natural drying

As we have seen, wet hair stretches more easily than dry hair. During most drying processes the hair is stretched into shape and position and dried into this form. Elastic recoil is delayed when the hair is dried and remains in this shape until the hair is made wet again, either when shampooed or as moisture is absorbed from the atmosphere, when it returns to its natural shape and direction.

When drying naturally, the hair remains in its unstretched state, having been gently put into shape and dried undisturbed either without heat or by applying radiant heat.

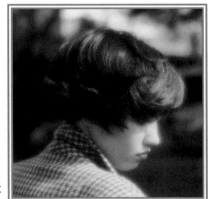

Figure 12.8 Finger dried hair

Setting hair

Setting is a technique used for styling the hair and reforming the shape of the hair temporarily. Hair is hygroscopic – it allows moisture to penetrate and enables us to reshape the hair when wet. By using various styling equipment and products you can transform the hair into a different shape by drying it in its newly formed position. However, this is only temporary as there are no chemicals involved to change the hair permanently.

The setting and curling techniques available today are creative and innovative as there is so much available to the stylist in terms of products and equipment that allow you to mould and change the shape of the hair to create a number of different textures on all types of hair.

Setting principles

Like blow drying, setting is a method of temporarily forming wet hair into a new shape then drying it. Hair structure is both elastic and flexible. As the hair is curled or shaped it is bent under tension into the shape of the roller or setting tool. In the case of a curler, the hair is stretched on the outer side of the curve and compressed on the inner side. If it is dried in the new position the curl will be retained. This happens because the hydrogen and salt bonds between the keratin chains are broken. The hair is then moved into its new temporary position. The stronger disulphide bonds remain unbroken; this is known as beta keratin.

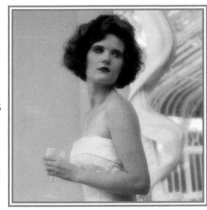

Hair is hygroscopic and able to retain moisture. As hair absorbs moisture the rearranged keratin chains loosen or relax into their previous shape and position. Hair that is in its natural unstretched shape is known as alpha keratin. This is why the humidity (content of moisture in the air) determines how long the curl shape is retained.

Figure 12.9

Setting techniques

Curling the hair

There are many types of methods and rollers that can be used to create a number of effects when setting and dressing the hair. They may need additional heat to dry the hair – note, these electrical appliances must be handled and used according to the manufacturer's instructions (see Unit G1). These include fan-assisted hooded hairdryers that the client sits underneath, rollerballs and climazones; these use infra-radiation.

Types of rollers include:

- Foam rollers, e.g. foam or cloth stems for spiral setting for curly, tight, loose, textured or spiral effects. Used on longer hair. (See Figure 12.10.)
- Velcro rollers, e.g. self-fixing rollers for a softer set on semi-damp hair or partial set for lift and body. Used on short to medium-length hair.
- Plastic rollers, e.g. rigid rollers that are secured with a pin used for first pli, a crisper set from wet to dry. These can be used on partialy dry hair for a softer look and can achieve all types of curl, waves and movements depending on the size of the roller and whether the hair is set on or off base. Used on all lengths of hair.
- Bendy wires, e.g. rubber-coated thin wires used for twisting and wrapping the hair around for alternative curls and twists. Used on medium to long hair.

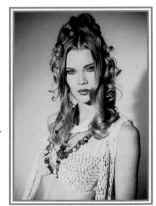

Heated appliances

- Electrically heated rollers can give a softer finish that is not crisp in its curl movement. These can be used for partial setting and full head of hair setting. Used on all hair lengths.

Figure 12.10

- Curlers for winding the hair down into a dome and snapping down to lock the hair into place giving an intermingled twist and soft curls. Used on medium to longer hair.
- Curling tongs are thermostatically controlled and are used on dry hair for curling, giving direction and spiral tonging. They come in various sizes and diameters.
- Flat irons or straighteners are used on dry hair and flatten the hair straight. These are thermostatically controlled.
- Crimping irons are used for crimping the hair and can be used on various lengths.
- Waving irons are used for waving the hair giving different sizes of wave variations.

Review Questions

1   Which bonds, located within the hair's cortex, are broken down and then reformed during the blow-dry process?

2   How much styling mousse is normally required when styling hair?

3   What effect will moisture have upon the finished hairstyle?

4   Which factors will affect your choice of styling technique to be used?

5   How may height be achieved in the hairstyle through blow drying?

6   When blow drying, how is a smooth effect achieved?

7   Which blow dryer attachment should be used when scrunch-drying hair?

8   What styling product should be used to help achieve separation and definition in a finished hairstyle?

9   What may be the result of applying too much gloss spray to the hair?

ACTIVITY

Outcome 1

- Describe the physical effects of drying the hair on the hair structure.
- Describe the effect humidity has on the hair structure.
- State how and when to use drying and styling equipment safely.
- Explain how the incorrect use of heat can affect the hair and scalp.
- Describe the current techniques for drying and styling the hair.
- Outline the Control of Substances Hazardous to Health Regulations 1992 (including subsequent amendments) and explain how they relate to styling and dressing products.
- State why it is important to check electrical equipment prior to use.

Outcome 2

- Describe the physical effects setting has on the hair structure.
- Describe the effect humidity has on the hair structure.

- *List the different types of equipment available for setting and dressing hair.*

- *Explain how and when to use setting equipment safely.*

- *State how the incorrect use of heat can affect the hair and scalp.*

- *Describe the current techniques for dressing and setting the hair.*

- *Outline the Control of Substances Hazardous to Health Regulations 1992 (including subsequent amendments) and explain how they relate to styling and dressing products.*

- *State why it is important to check electrical equipment prior to use.*

13 UNIT H26 STYLE AND DRESS LONG HAIR

1 Maintain effective and safe methods of working when styling long hair

2 Creatively dress long hair

CHAPTER CONTENTS

- *Work Safely When Dressing Long Hair*
- *Vertical Rolls*
- *Horizontal Rolls*
- *Combination Rolls*
- *Chignons*
- *Plaits*
- *Twists and Knots*
- *Added Hair*
- *Ornamentation*
- *Development Activities*
- *Additional Information*
- *Activity*

Introduction

Dressing long hair can be very exciting but it can also be quite daunting if you do not know how to approach your desired hairstyle. Through experience I have learnt to master the technique purely by following the three Ps – planning, patience and practice.

Most stylists tend to steer clear of this service because they don't feel confident or are afraid the end result is not what the client will want. Long hair is extremely fashionable these days and there seem to be more and more special events that the clients want to attend with a different or special look. If learners are encouraged to practise and experiment while studying they tend to go from strength to strength, mastering the techniques below.

Working with long hair is very much like cutting. You learn the techniques, build your confidence, work with various types of hair and design shapes to balance the head and body shapes. Study your craft, look in the media for shapes emerging and trends. Take it a step further by looking in art galleries, etc, to stimulate your own artistic ability.

This is an advanced level of hairdressing and you should be developing looks that are balanced and creative. Photograph your work. Look and see how your work is developing over a period of time.

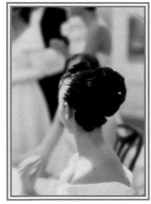

Figure 13.1

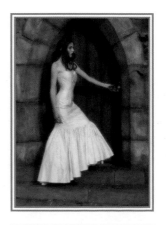

Figure 13.2

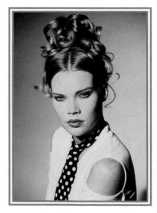

Figure 13.3

Make notes of what you feel worked well and why. Carry a pencil and paper around and sketch shapes that interest you and that you can develop in your work. Enjoy yourself and master your craft.

Work safely when dressing long hair

There are many techniques available and a variety of tools and equipment that can be used when dressing long hair.

- It is important that you carry out a consultation prior to starting the client's hair for any contraindications and also to agree the end result (see Unit G9).
- You need to prepare tools and equipment so that you can work safely and methodically.
- If using hot irons, straighteners, heated rollers, crimping irons, etc, ensure they are not left switched on as there is a risk of someone burning themselves.
- Do not leave trailing flexes around and disconnect when not in use.
- Do not open hair grips by putting them in your mouth.
- Use grips and hair fasteners safely ensuring the client's comfort.
- Heat and humidity can affect the hair and can cause dryness and damage if not used correctly.
- Sterilise your tools and equipment using disinfectants, autoclaves and ultraviolet sterilisers.
- Keep the area you work in clean and tidy.
- Keep client records in a secure place, remembering the Data Protection Act. For more information see Unit G9.
- Use products safely, and read and follow manufacturer's guidelines for safe use.
- Clean up spillages immediately.
- Ensure the client is comfortable at all times, especially if she needs to sit under hairdryers, etc.

Vertical rolls

Other names associated with this look are a pleat, French pleat and thumb roll.

The vertical roll has always been a popular way to dress hair. It can be adapted in many ways depending on the look you want to achieve.

Look Desired	Interpretation
Classic	Smooth, sleek, simple, elegant, timeless appeal
Fashionable	Reflecting the latest trends shown on the catwalks, magazines and in the media, commercial
Avant-garde	Forerunner of fashion, ahead of its time, over-exaggerated, utilised as a medium creatively
Historic	Period looks reflecting an era, e.g. nineteenth century, 1980s

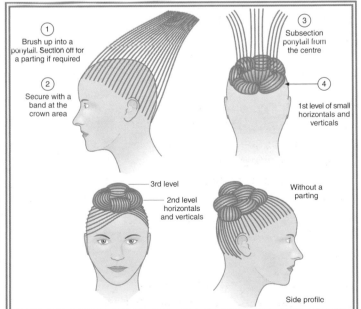

Figure 13.4 Vertical and horizontal rolls

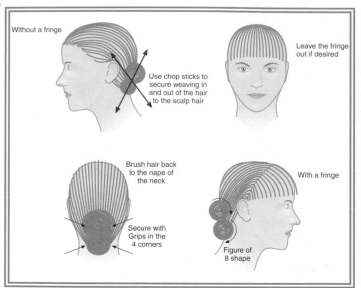

Figure 13.5 Chiffons

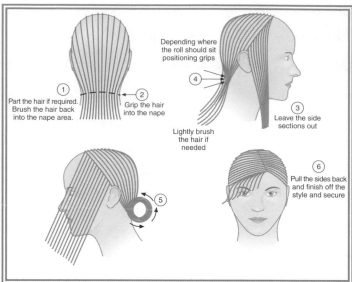

Figure 13.6 Horizontal rolls

Techniques used to dress the vertical roll

Technique	Preparation	Reason	Look
Directional dry hair setting	Heated rollers placed in the direction of the vertical roll in dry hair that may have products applied, e.g. conditioner, styling products	Smooths the cuticle of the hair, gives lift, body and movement in the desired direction. Products used to personalise finished look and help secure hair	Classic, fashionable, historic. More finished, can be softer if required
Directional wet hair setting	Wet hair set on large, medium or small rollers in the direction of the vertical roll depending on the amount of curl needed. Hair may have products applied, e.g. conditioner, styling products	Firmer finish, smooths the cuticle, gives curl, body and movement. Can last longer if grips have been secured correctly as hair is dressed up. Products used to personalise finished look and help secure hair	Wavy, smooth, curly. More finished classic, fashionable, historic, textured
Partial setting, wet setting or dry hair	Section hair into sub-sections. Set the area needing movement, body and control. Use products appropriate to wet or dry setting and the desired look	If you want some areas flat then do not set. If you need more control and movement of some areas then set the hair	Commercial, fashionable
Blow dry straight	Wash the hair the day before. If washing the hair on the day then use a styling lotion to help smooth the hair and control it	The hair is easier to handle and not so slippery. Creates a more natural look	Commercial, fashionable

Dry heat setting technique using heated rollers

Use the correct products to try to help control the hair.

Section the hair into sub sections.

Wet hair setting technique using rollers on wet hair then drying the hair under a hairdryer

Use the correct products to try to help control the hair.

Section the hair into sub-sections.

Partial hair setting technique using heated rollers

Use the correct products to try to help control the hair.

Section the hair into sub-sections.

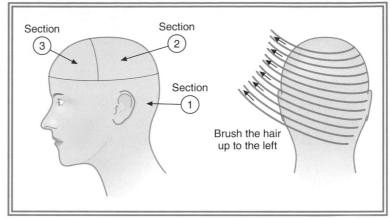

Figure 13.6a Sectioning the hair for a vertical roll

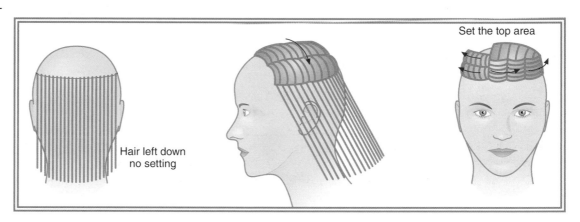

Figure 13.6c Partial hair setting

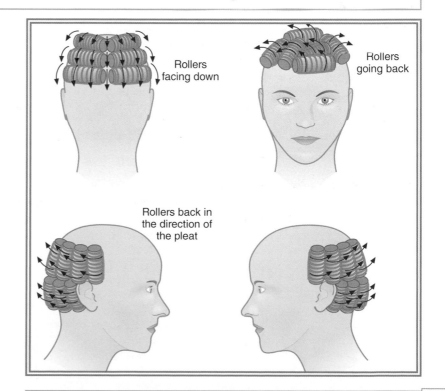

Figure 13.6b Vertical roll setting

1 Backcombing gives the hair body to help secure the pins so that they do not slip out easily. It will give the client's hair body if it is fine.

2 Once the hair is backcombed, smooth the top of the hair with a soft brush, being careful not to take the backcombing out. Lightly brush the hair from right to left and slightly upwards.

3 Place the grips upwards and put in a line from the nape to the crown area, or criss-cross the grips if preferred. This will secure them, avoiding accidental removal. However, they can then be difficult to remove or change their position part way through the dressing.

4 Now brush the hair from the opposite side, again lightly on the top from left to right. Twist the hair up and fold the ends inside. Make sure the hair is still smooth and shiny, allowing the backcombing to remain to secure the grips inside the fold and onto the scalp.

5 You need to have decided which finish you would like and dress the hair according to the desired shape, e.g. fashionable, classic or avant-garde.

6 Now backcomb the two side sections. Today's fashion replicates images such as Mohicans. This shape can interpret the Mohican by adapting the vertical roll from the nape to the forehead. Shape and mould the texture of the hair.

7 Smooth the hair from the side and smooth over the vertical line, making sure the style is balanced and complimentary to the head shape.

8 Use hairspray if you need to control the hair.

9 Look at the balance, using mirrors to help you.

10 Decide now whether to put the hair at the front, on the side or style it straight back from the face. You could backcomb the hair and make it high.

11 You can split the sections into smaller sections if you find it more manageable.

12 You can separate the hair and make it very classic or spike the hair.

Horizontal rolls

Horizontal rolls are rolls across the head. This technique can be used in a variety of ways. The look can be very striking when used to emphasise the contours of the head shape. The three main areas used to accentuate the head shape are the nape, the crown and the forehead.

The nape (the lowest point of the head)

1 Decide on a parting if required. Section the sides from ear to ear and across the crown area.

2 Leave these sections out.

3 Brush the hair back to the nape area. At this point you can backcomb for body or just brush the hair flat to the head. Secure the hair in the nape by gripping or by securing in a band, keeping it as close to the scalp as possible. N.B. Head position is important here. If the head is too far forward it can make the roll baggy. Decide if you want the roll tight or baggy, low or high and then secure. Do not put the grips in your mouth to open them as it is unprofessional and unhygienic.

4 Once the hair is secure bring each of the sides back to cover the band by wrapping around, or leave the sides out to personalise the hairstyle, depending on what you want to achieve.

5 Roll the hair upwards secure with grips.

6 Finish using ornamentation or products to define and exaggerate hair shapes.

The crown (the highest point of the head)

1 Use the same technique as above, this time securing hair on the crown area. Move the roll to various points on the crown and look at the profile.

2 This is a great style for weddings, as tiaras and veils are supported by the roll.

The forehead (furthest point forward)

Directions:

1 *Again use the same technique as above but place the roll at the forehead. Move the roll around to complement the face shape. Look at the profile. Dress with and without a fringe.*

These styles are easy to produce and very effective. They can be developed using fresh flowers, ornamentation, etc. You can combine the rolls by putting one on top of the other. You can place a roll in the nape and forehead giving a 50s feel.

Use supports that can be bought from any hairdressing suppliers or most chemist's. This enables you to roll the hair around and support the roll from the inside. They come in various sizes and colours. Alternatively, make your own supports out of crepe hair, tights, etc.

Combination rolls – vertical and horizontal

Other names used for this style are barrel curls and hair up.

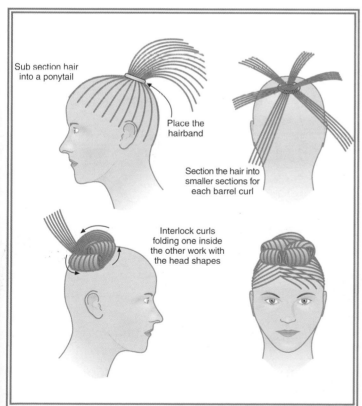

Sub section hair into a ponytail

Place the hairband

Section the hair into smaller sections for each barrel curl

Interlock curls folding one inside the other work with the head shapes

Figuer 13.6d Combination rolls

This is a combination of rolls, usually smaller and interlocking. Again you can create a variety of looks.

Directions:

1 *Using the shape of the head, decide on the look and the occasion.*

2 *Plan your shape.*

3 *Subsection the hair to make it more manageable, e.g. ponytails.*

4 *Brush the hair into place.*

5 *Place the hair in a band.*

6 *Section the hair again, working out how many curls you want and where they should be, e.g. five curls at the bottom, three on the next level, one at the top.*

7 *Grip each curl individually and build by gripping one section at the base and then grip again securing the curl, being careful not to show the grips. The great thing with this technique is that you can make the hairstyle as high as you want, as low as you want, as wide or as narrow as you want.*

8 *Finish off the hairstyle with products or ornamentation as required.*

If the hair is not long enough, use a hairpiece with grips and attach the base.

By setting the ponytail or hairpiece you will give a smoother finished look and it will help to curl the hair around into the roll/curl.

You can use this technique to produce softer loose curls instead of horizontal and vertical rolls. They can be placed around the head, nape, crown, back of the head to symmetrical or asymmetrical shapes.

Chignons

This is a very simple technique that can be mastered using the flat part of the hand.

Directions:

1 *Brush the hair down into the nape of the neck.*

2 *Hold the hair in the centre of the nape and wrap the hair around four fingers. Hold the fingers out and flat.*

3 Turn the hand anti-clockwise all the way around until you are pointing at the 6.30 p.m. position.

4 Pull the hair through until you can't see the ends.

5 The centre will form a figure 8 shape. Secure this with grips into the four corners, using chopsticks or pins.

Plaits

Plaiting has always been a popular way to dress hair and can be extremely creative.

Start by using two strands, picking up hair each time from the scalp on the opposite side. If you want the plait to sit on the scalp you will need to bend the head so that the area you are plaiting is in line with your hands. The hand position is important here as the plait can become baggy if your hands are held too high.

Watch to make sure the plait is even; again head position and tension is important here.

Add ornamentation, flowers or ribbons depending on the occasion.

Leave the ends out or fold, tuck in and grip onto the scalp for a more finished look. Leave the plaits in overnight for a crimped look the following day.

Once you move on to five-stem plaits you will need another operator to help.

With five-stem plaits you start with three stems then build up to five or more, usually an uneven number.

1 Start with three stems, pick up from the outside, working under and over towards the centre.

2 Cross the centre over.

3 Pick up from the other side and repeat working into the centre.

Twists and knots

A great and simple way to tie hair up, giving it shape and texture.

Plan where you want the hair to be placed to create the desired shape and pre-set if required depending on look to be created. Figure 13.8 shows hair that has been previously set with heated rollers. Once the rollers have been taken out one section has been tied to the other. Some of the curls have been left out at the ends. Again ornamentation, postiche or flowers can be added for the finished look.

Twisting can be carried out on the scalp or you can subsection the hair, placing the twists exactly where you want them.

This is again very simple and very effective. Secure the twists with grips or pins. Make sure the grips are the correct colour and hide them under the twist. Fine pins are useful – the end can be bent, 'fish hooked', to stop them sliding out of the hair too easily.

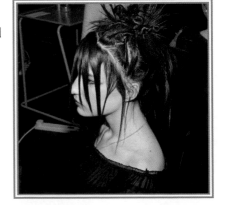

Figure 13.7 Twists

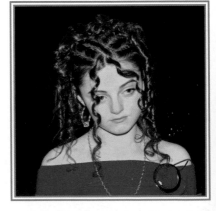

Figure 13.8 Twists and curls

Added hair

This is a great way to really be creative.

You can buy added hair from numerous places, e.g. specialist hair and wig suppliers (wholesale and retail), trade fairs and even some charity shops, etc.

You can buy monofibre, synthetic and real hair in all shapes and sizes on all types of bases. Real hair needs careful attention as it can knot up easily. Read the manufacturer's instruction for cleaning and styling. Don't shampoo unless recommended by the manufacturer.

Monofibre is treated differently to real hair but again follow manufacturer's instructions for styling and cleaning. Usually warm water with a mild detergent is used for cleaning followed by a conditioner (can be fabric conditioner). Remember this is artificial hair so do not use curling tongs as it can melt the monofibre.

Hairpieces

These come on various shaped bases in different sizes and in different lengths and textures. The most commonly used are machine-made bases with combs or clips for hair-up styles – half head pieces that you can attach at the crown area to give volume and length, fringes and ponytails. There is usually a colour chart to choose your hairpiece from. They can be attached by grips but some hairpieces have clips or combs already fixed on the base. There is a fantastic choice these days when buying hair – a wide selection of colours, textures and weights.

Weight is very important when buying a hairpiece as some can be too heavy for the client's scalp, making it uncomfortable to wear. Make sure it has a base that you can easily attach.

You can prepare the hairpiece by setting and dressing, e.g. barrel curls.

Extensions

You can get real hair extensions or synthetic. You can extend the hair length, give more volume or add colour, matching the colours or textures to suit the client's hair.

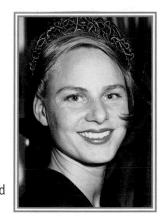

There are various techniques used when adding hair extensions or weave-ins. Monofibre is attached by using four stem braids at the base then securing by creating a seal with a heated gun. Bonding is sometimes used to stop the extension from slipping out. Real hair extensions can be attached using bonding solutions. They can be quite time consuming to apply but, if applied correctly, last for up to three months.

Care must be given when dressing the hair with extensions so as not to break or pull on the extension. There is usually a bedding-in period, which allows for the heat from the head to expand and contract the extension, during which time a few extensions may be lost. It is important to follow the maintenance programme to get the most out of the extensions and keep them looking good. Special products and tools can be used to keep the extensions from falling out.

Figure 13.9 Crepe hair

Extensions are great for adding vibrant and natural highlights to the hair as the colour doesn't fade.

Crepe hair

Crepe hair is great for building and creating weird and avant-garde shapes. It is also used for support and padding for theatrical and historical looks. It comes in various colours and lengths and is made from hair and/or wool that has been frizzed by weaving around strings and permanently fixing.

Ornamentation

There is a great variety of ornamentation available from wholesalers, chemists, departmental stores and accessory shops. Ornamentation can dress up the simplest of hairstyles to make it look fashionable, classic, historical or avant-garde. Depending on how creative you are, you can even design your own ornamentation. Again, careful planning and preparation to secure the ornamentation needs to be given to make sure it stays in place.

Decorative diamante tiaras and clips, combs and artificial flowers can also be used.

Points to remember

- Always make a plan of the style you are going to create.

- Break it down into smaller sections to make it manageable.

- Depending on the hairstyle, setting the hair will allow the ends to curl around easily and smooth the cuticle, giving shine.

- Make sure the hair is balanced. Look at the hairstyle from different angles and alter if necessary.

- Backcomb the hair to support the grips.

- Spray the hair lightly. Do not over product the hair.

- Use the natural fall to help you to decide if you are going to use a side parting.

- Use the right tools for the job.

Development activities

- Try out the hairstyles listed above.

- Photograph these hairstyles.

- Make up a portfolio to see how your work is developing.

- Once you feel the end result is as you want, make up a long hair style book for your clients to see.

- Use a combination of your work and photographs from magazines.

- Separate these photographs into sculptured looks, bridal hair, special occasion hair, etc.

Additional information

Useful websites

Website Addresses	Content
www.habia.org.uk	Hairdressing and Beauty Industry Authority. Downloads available including references to other websites
www.bbc-safety.co.uk	Free advice on health and safety
www.lookfantastic.com	Professional hairdressing products and advice
www.laurandp.co.uk	Educational publications for development of professional hairdressing
www.scott999.fsnet.co.uk	Hairdressing product information
www.nexus.com	Range of hairdressing products
www.tigi.co.uk	Range of hairdressing products
www.schwarzkopf.com	Range of hairdressing products
www.loreal.com	Range of hairdressing products

Magazines and journals

- *Hairdressers Journal*
- *Creative Head*
- *Estetica/Cutting Edge*
- *Black Beauty and Hair*

Book

Patrick Cameron's *Long Hairdressing*

Not only will this build your confidence but it will also help you to gain assessment if you are working towards your NVQ Level 3 Hairdressing Unit 26. If you are studying The Modern Apprenticeship Framework, then you will need to complete the following outcomes.

ACTIVITY

Outcomes 1 and 2

Make a presentation on the legal responsibilities and the impact of legislation on hairdressing to include health and safety and client confidentiality. You should use two charts showing (1) the links between client information and legal requirements and (2) safety issues in the salon with particular reference to the styling and finishing process.

Outcomes 3, 4, 5 and 6

An evaluation, via a case study, of an observation of a senior colleague at work with four clients with different styling and finishing needs. The case study should be in written or oral format and should include reference to the client records, product and equipment selection and critical influencing factors that guided their choice. The candidate must include a chart showing the correct understanding of client preparation and treatment, specifically:

- *amounts of styling and finishing products used*
- *the sequence of products and equipment used, including timescales*
- *styling techniques used*
- *health and safety considerations.*

Outcomes 2, 4

Complete the activity listed above on long hair. Evidence from additional information must be included, e.g. hairstyles from the internet.

14 UNIT H27 CREATE A VARIETY OF LOOKS USING A COMBINATION OF CUTTING TECHNIQUES

1 Maintain effective and safe methods when cutting hair

2 Cut hair to create a variety of looks for women

CHAPTER CONTENTS

- *Haircutting Tools*
- *Recap*
- *Foundation Techniques – One-length Bob*
- *Foundation Techniques – Long One Length*
- *Square Layers*
- *Rounded Layers*
- *Graduated Layers*

- *Review*
- *Haircutting Shapes*
- *Assessing the Head for Cutting*
- *Basic Guidelines when Cutting Hair*
- *Combination Haircuts*
- *Additional Information*
- *Activity*

Introduction

Cutting hair is one of the most important of all the hairdressing skills. A good haircut, skilfully executed, can transform the most mediocre head of hair into something special. To cut hair proficiently the hairdresser must be aware of where and how the length and bulk (weight) need to be removed in order to create a desirable shape with good line and balance. Each head of hair differs in some way and each haircut should be carefully cut to emphasise any good points and minimise any defects. Remember that a good haircut is the basis for all good hairdressing. When a blow dry or set has dropped from the hair, all that remains is the shape of the haircut!

Haircutting tools

These include:

- scissors
- razors
- clippers
- combs
- neck brush.

Scissors

These may be obtained in a variety of lengths and weights. The choice of length and weight is entirely up to the individual but it is important that the scissors feel comfortable. When purchasing a new pair of scissors, test them first by holding between the thumb and the third finger, as this is how they should be held

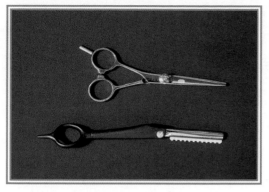

Figure 14.1 Scissors

Figure 14.2 Razors

when cutting the hair, they should feel as if they are an extension of the fingers. Hairdressing scissors should only be used for cutting hair. Using them for cutting string, paper, etc, will blunt the blades very quickly and blunt blades will tear the hair.

Plain straight edged scissors

Used for normal cutting, including both club and taper cutting techniques. The longer blade lengths are used for scissor over comb techniques.

Very fine serrated edge scissors

The serrations hold the hair in place along the blade when cutting. They can be used for all cutting techniques except when slither cutting the hair, e.g. taper cutting or slide cutting. In this case the finely serrated edge of the scissors tends to drag on the hair and does not cut it as cleanly as the straight-edged scissors.

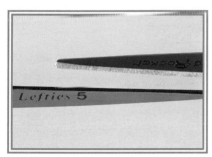

Figure 14.3 Smooth blade and blade with micro-serrations

Wide-spaced serrated edge scissors

These are known as aesculap scissors. Either one blade or both blades are serrated to allow a limited amount of hair only to be cut. This type of scissors is usually used to remove bulk or weight from the hair, e.g. thinning. However, there are many different types of aesculap scissors, some designed to remove more hair than others. The choice of aesculap depends upon the required result and also the stylist's personal preference. They are usually used on dry hair; if used on wet hair extra care must be taken not to remove too much bulk, as the wet hairs tend to stick together.

The razor

The guarded razor has a replaceable blade, which is protected by a metal guard and is attached to a fixed or movable handle. It is known either as a 'shaper' razor or it is shaped like an open razor, and is used in preference to the open razor by most present-day salons. An open or cut-throat razor requires far more care in use than a safety razor. For more information see Unit H19.

Clippers

There are two types of clippers: hand clippers and electric clippers. Both types consist of two blades with sharp-edged teeth. One blade remains fixed while the other moves across it. The distance between the blade teeth determines the closeness of the haircut. Used in men's and ladies' haircutting to produce very short haircuts. For more information see Unit H21.

Combs

Cutting combs have two sizes of teeth, spaced to allow easy taking of sections and combing the hair when wet or dry. The comb should not have sharp edges that may cut either you or the client and should be rigid enough to comb through a section without flexing too much. Combs for scissor over comb technique are more pliable and allow the hair to be cut nearer to the scalp, for example, short graduation, short back and sides, and shingle, etc.

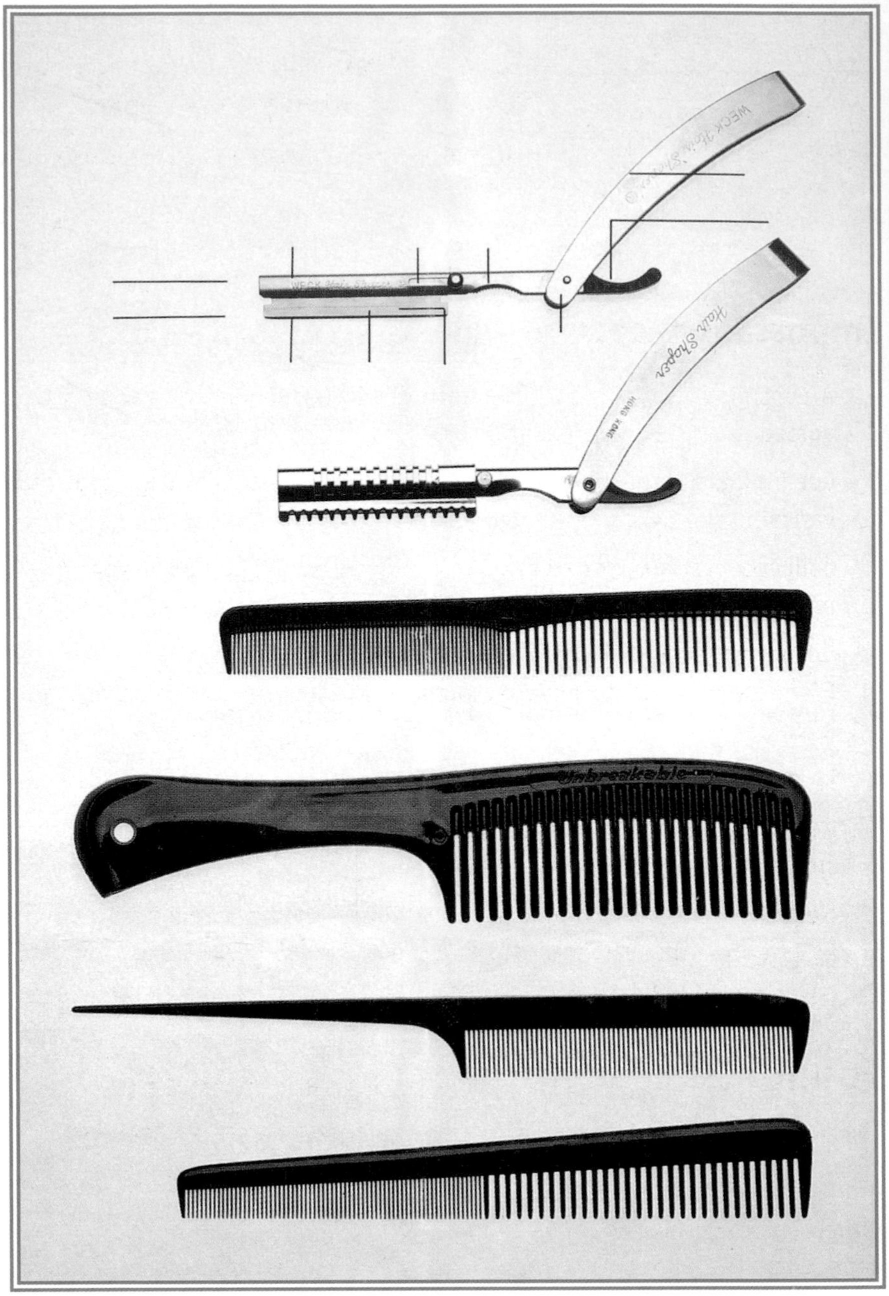

Neck brush

These are used to remove the loose hairs from the face and the neck after cutting the hair. They are made from bristle, nylon or a combination of both. They can be used with talcum powder sprinkled onto the brush to aid the removal of wet hair from the skin.

Recap

Before cutting hair at this level you need to recap on what you already know and ensure you have learnt your foundation cutting skills well. This level of hair cutting usually requires you to combine these skills and then extend your experience further to incorporate personalising techniques. This is crucial to the success of the cut today. This combination and how a haircut is interpreted gives the hair stylist their own identity and is why a client wants them to be their personal stylist.

More and more clients are aware of what is required for a good haircut as there is a lot of information available in the media and press. How many times have you heard them say, 'I want my hair to look like that celebrity'?

You should be able to look at the hairstyle and, through your knowledge and expertise, interpret the cut to suit and balance the client. You may be cutting the client's hair for a number of reasons, whether it is classic, fashionable for a film or production or just to make them look good.

Figure 14.4 Top to bottom: Replacement blade open razor; open razor with safety guards; all purpose comb; large-tooth comb; tail comb; hair shaping comb

The following is a guide to help you recap and build on your existing knowledge. I hope you find it useful. Remember: you can never stop learning. Even very talented stylists need to stop, every now and again, and look at what they are doing and how other hair professionals are performing. You need to look at ways you can improve.

Let's recap! The table below is common ground in terms of looks desired. If you can think of any others please add them to the list and interpret. Remember: hairdressing is continuously changing and that is what makes it so exciting.

Look Desired	Interpretation
Classic	Smooth, sleek, simple, elegant, timeless appeal
Fashionable	Reflecting the latest trends shown on the catwalks, magazines and in the media, commercial
Avant-garde	Forerunner of fashion, ahead of its time, over exaggerated, utilised as a medium creatively

Important factors to consider prior to cutting

● A consultation must be carried out prior to any hairdressing service to ensure the correct results are achieved and agreed with the client (see Unit G9).

● Cutting hair is technical and using the correct method is important as every head of hair, shape of skull and hair type varies.

● Collect a portfolio of hairstyles to show your client so you can agree with the client what they want and as a professional what you would advise. Some clients know exactly what they want and others need to be guided. The portfolio supports effective communication.

● For these reasons you must take special care to consult the client and match the technique most suited to the desired look.

● Look at the facial features and body shape to balance the haircut so that it is complementary to the client.

● Agree a hair maintenance programme so that the client will rebook their next appointment to keep their hairstyle in shape.

● Help the client by showing them how to get the best from their haircut using the correct products and equipment, and by offering other services to complement the cut, e.g. colour, blow drying, etc.

● Use the correct tools for the job.

Foundation techniques – one-length bob

The one-length bob is also known as one length, Halo and Pageboy.

A one-length bob is a haircut without any graduation or layers. The haircut is formed by letting the hair fall naturally to form a one-length outline. The one-length bob has always been a popular way to cut hair. It can be adapted in many ways depending on the look you want to achieve. It can be square, 'A' line, rounded or halo with or without a parting, with or without a fringe. Body position is crucial to the success of the cut. Some stylists like to cut the hair while the client is sitting down. Other stylists like their clients to stand up, especially if the hair is below shoulder length. You have to consider the client's comfort, but need to cut the hair as close to the skin as possible.

Ensure the client is sitting or standing straight with their head tilted slightly forward when working the back sections. If you do not, you may end up with some graduation or the hairstyle being lopsided.

The hair is usually best cut using the client's natural parting unless specified otherwise. Use small sections and ensure you can see the guideline. Do not lift the hair, over direct or use too much tension. Sometimes if you are cutting a child's hair it is not safe to cut against the skin. Use your discretion as you may need to cut holding the hair and compensate.

Observe the growth patterns and how the head contours change as you work through each step. Ears protrude – try not to catch them when combing and always release the tension to allow the hair to fall naturally.

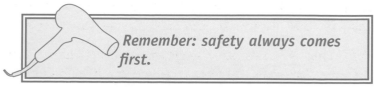

Remember: safety always comes first.

Techniques used to cut the one-length bob

Technique	Preparation	Reason	Look
One-length bob above the shoulders but below the hairline. Cut on wet hair. Decide the outline shape Section the hair into manageable sections *Step by step technique* ***Figure 14.5***	Prepare by wetting the hair down Section the hair using sectioning clips Use a cutting comb (preferably with wide teeth so as not to use too much tension) Use products if desired *Step by step technique* 1 Section hair as in Figure 14.5 2 The section line should reflect the cutting line 3 Cut the hair by combing it downwards into its natural fall on the neck 4 Place the scissors blade flat underneath the hair to ensure you do not cut the skin and close the top blade to cut the hair to the desired length and shape 5 Cut one side then repeat section by section alternating from side to side. Make sure you can see the guideline 6 Leave the crown area until last and when the hair is dry to avoid graduation 7 Move to the side section 8 Again make sure the head is tilted e.g. left side, tilt head to the right away from you. Keep the chin up slightly 9 Section as in Figure 14.6. Cut the hair as near to the skin as possible 10 Look at the information above relating to ears 11 Continue taking small sections until you reach the natural parting	Makes the hair more manageable To ensure the cutting section is controllable To control the hair without using too much tension Products control the hair So you do not cut the client To ensure you check the balance, symmetrical or asymmetrical, depending on the look When hair is wet the crown area falls flat. When it is dry it sometimes springs up unevenly and could cause graduation To get the hair to turn under, the more you tilt the head the more reverse graduation will occur. The top layer will be slightly longer To avoid uneven outline To ensure you keep to the guideline and the outline	Classic, fashionable, historic More finished, can be softer if required

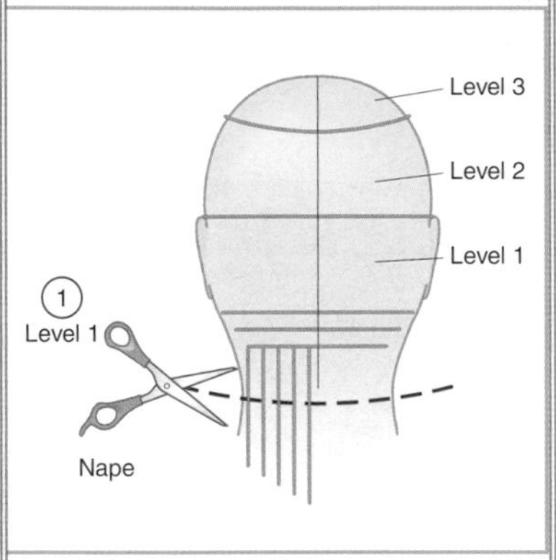

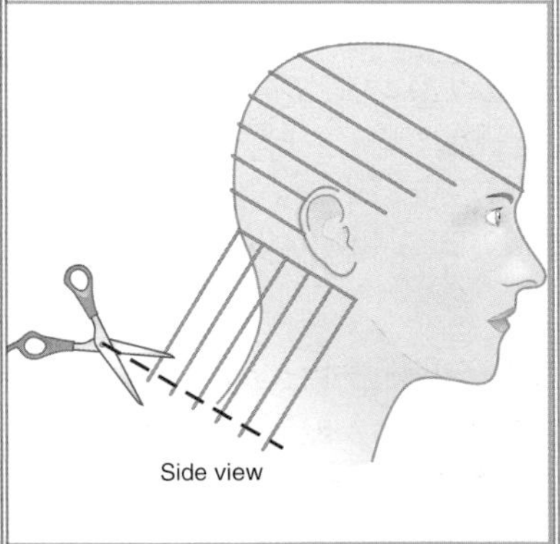

Figure 14.6

Technique	Preparation	Reason	Look
Figure 14.7 *Figure 14.8*	12 Repeat this for the other side (see Figure 14.7) 13 Make sure you use a guideline to ensure that the haircut is balanced 14 At this stage the haircut is almost complete. You now need to look at your client with head upright and from all different angles 15 Comb the hair through and rough dry freehand. Cut the crown area now to complete the cut 16 Get your client to shake her hair thoroughly and check the hair is sitting properly. Cut any odd hairs that fall below the outline	To achieve balance To allow the crown to spring up into its natural fall and avoid cutting too short Hair stretches when wet. Drying the hair and letting it fall into its new shape will let you see the precision of the cut more clearly	
Create this bob into a variety of cuts	Personalise this haircut by using a variety of techniques – slide cutting, razor cutting, undercutting, cropping, texturising, layering, graduating. See advanced cutting techniques at the end of this section		
One length halo completely round in shape with no corners	The same technique for one length using horizontal sections but this time a rounded perimeter with fringe. Therefore Section lines are rounded and combined into the netural fall forward.	Do not over direct or use tension as this may cause graduation. Ideally cut on the skin. Ideal length directly beneath the nape hairline and underneath the ear lobe	

Foundation techniques – long one length

This style is also known as one length, square one length and rounded one length.

A long one length is a haircut without any graduations or layers below the shoulders. The haircut is formed by letting the hair fall naturally to form a one-length outline. The one length has always been a popular way to cut hair. It can be adapted in many ways depending on the look you want to achieve, e.g. square or rounded, with or without a fringe.

Again, body position is crucial to the success of the haircut. Some stylists like to cut the client's hair while the client stands. This enables them to get a precision line falling naturally below the shoulders. The main emphasis with this haircut is to try to cut the client's hair as close to the body as possible, thus preventing graduation. If you have to cut the client's hair through your fingers, then you may need the head to be tilted forward slightly more than normal, thus creating reverse graduation.

Point to remember: if a client is standing, check to make sure that she is not bending her knee or standing for too long. Standing not only gives a precision line but is far easier for the stylist as it prevents them from having to bend too much, thus causing backache. Cutting stools can be used but beware that the chair or towel, etc, does not obstruct the natural fall on to the body.

Ensure the client is sitting or standing straight, depending on the stylist's choice. Try to use a guideline, e.g. shoulder blade, so that when you cut the opposite side the haircut is fairly balanced. Visual checks using mirrors and standing away from the haircut at intervals will enable you to ensure the haircut is not lopsided or going off at an angle.

The hair is usually best cut using the natural parting, unless the client specifies otherwise. However, as the hair is longer the weight of the hair will hold the haircut in the desired parting, unlike a bob. If the hair is short it tends to bounce up into the natural parting. This depends on the natural density of the hair.

Again use small sections. Always make sure you can see your guideline. If you lose your guideline, stop and go back until you can find it.

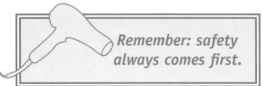

Remember: safety always comes first.

Do not lift the hair, over direct or use too much tension. Sometimes if you are cutting a child's hair it is not safe to cut on the skin. Use your discretion as you may need to cut holding the hair and compensate.

Observe the growth patterns and how the head contours change as you work through each step. Ears protrude – be careful not to catch them when combing, and always release the tension to allow the hair to fall naturally.

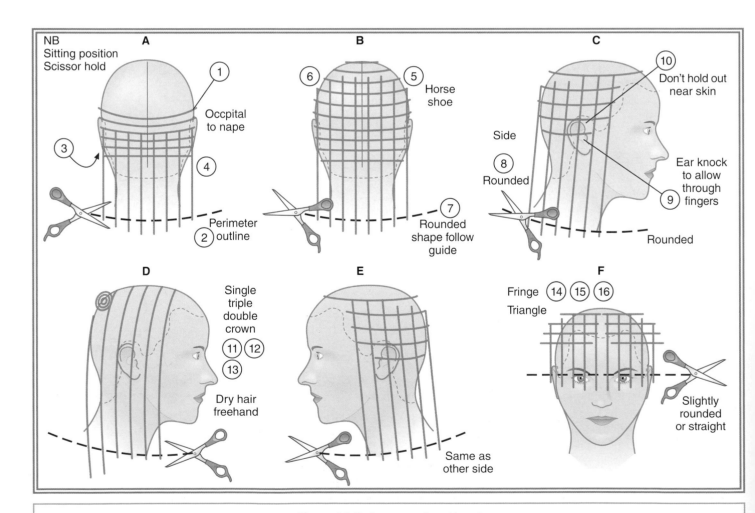

Figure 14.9 Long one length cut

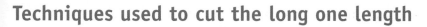

Techniques used to cut the long one length

Technique	Preparation	Reason	Look
Long one length below the shoulders. Cut on wet or dry hair (preferably wet)			Classic, fashionable, historic. More finished, can be softer if required
Cut on wet hair	Prepare by wetting the hair down	Makes the hair more manageable	
Decide the outline shape. Section the hair into manageable sections	Section the hair using sectioning clips. Use a cutting comb (preferably with wide teeth so as not to use too much tension). Use products if desired	To ensure the cutting section is controllable To control the hair without using too much tension Products control the hair	
	1 Section hair as in Figure 14.9A		
	2 The section line should reflect the cutting line, e.g. square or round		
	3 Cut the hair by combing it downwards into its natural fall on the back (ensure the back is not too hollow and the shoulders are straight, the knees are not bent and the head is tilted slightly forward). At this stage you could get the client to balance themselves by holding on to something stable		
	4 Place the scissor blade flat to the client's back and open and close your thumb to cut the hair in a straight line (or slightly rounded, whatever you prefer)	So you do not cut the client's clothes, gown or towel. A cutting collar is advisable	
	For square one length when cutting the hair at the back, once you have the perimeter line comb the hair from the right to left to check the middle perimeter length and vice versa for the other side		
	5 Cut one side then repeat section by section, alternating from side to side. Make sure you can see the guideline	Ensure you check the balance to make sure the haircut is symmetrical (unless otherwise desired)	

Technique	Preparation	Reason	Look
	6 Leave cutting the crown area until last as the hair will be dry and will avoid graduation	When the hair is wet the crown area falls flat. When the hair is dry it sometimes springs up unevenly. Therefore it is safer to cut when dry	
	7 Move to the side section. At this point the head position changes depending on whether square one length or rounded one length is required ● For square one length, all the hair is cut behind the shoulders ● For rounded one length, the head position is as in point 7 onwards		
Rounded one length	8 Again, make sure the head position is lifted – raise the client's chin and tilt head away from the stylist. Keep chin raised	Remember to keep the chin raised to ensure that the hair is the same length all the way round. If the chin is tilted down you may cut the hair shorter at the front, thus leaving hair longer at the back	
	9 Section. Cut the hair as near to the skin as possible, following points 7 and 8.		
	10 Be careful not to catch the ears when combing, and always release the tension to allow the hair to fall naturally	This will avoid uneven outline	
	11 Continue taking small sections until you reach the natural parting	This will ensure you keep to the guideline and the outline	
	12 Repeat this for the other side, repeating from point 7 onwards		
	13 Make sure you use a guideline	This will ensure that the haircut is balanced	
	14 At this stage the haircut is almost complete. You now need to look at your client with the head up and from all different angles		
	15 Comb the hair through and rough dry. Cut the crown freehand	Rough drying will allow the crown to spring up into its natural fall and will avoid cutting the hair too short	
	16 Section the hair into a triangle, depending on the depth of fringe required	The triangle will be different on every client as it depends on the weight required, the shape of the forehead and the growth patterns	

Technique	Preparation	Reason	Look
	17 Section for a straight fringe. Pre-dampen the fringe at this point. Do not cut with tension and allow for the hair to shrink up as hair is elastic and can lose up to 30 per cent once it is dry	Cutting with too much tension if you have an uneven hairline will give you an uneven fringe. Freehand is far better, allowing the hair to dry partially. Ensure the client closes her eyes and make sure the scissors are held safely to avoid any accidents occurring	
	18 Take small sections, following the cutting pattern. Ensure you can always see your guideline		
	Fringes are extremely important to the haircut. The outline shape can be convex, concave, symmetrical, asymmetrical, layered, square or rounded depending on the client's wishes but remember this can change the balance of the whole haircut. It is up to the stylist to advise and guide the client for best results		
	19 When the cut is complete, blow dry as required then shake the head. Brush through and check the cut. Finish the cut freehand if required	Hair stretches when wet. Drying the hair and letting it fall into its new shape will let you see the precision of the cut more clearly	

Square layers

Square layers are also known as box layers, short layers, graduated layers and long layers.

Layering can be quite complex if you do not understand exactly what you want to achieve. The most important part of the consultation is assessing the client's head shape to get the length and balance required correct.

The haircut to be outlined is called a square layer. It is given this name because when the hair is blown directly away from the head it forms the shape of a box or square. This cut can be done at various lengths and will give a totally different look depending on the texture and density of the hair.

Usually the haircut starts from the shortest part, e.g. the side or the middle at the back. To make it easier we will go through this technique breaking the hair down into three levels. Level 1 starts from the nape of the neck to the occipital bone right round to the sides. Level 2 starts from where the first level finishes to just underneath the crown to the frontal area at the widest part of the head. Level 3 is the crown and frontal area and starts where the second level finishes.

Remember: Everybody's bone structure is different therefore the sections are important to be able to adapt the haircut to different head shapes. This ensures the haircut complements the head shape.

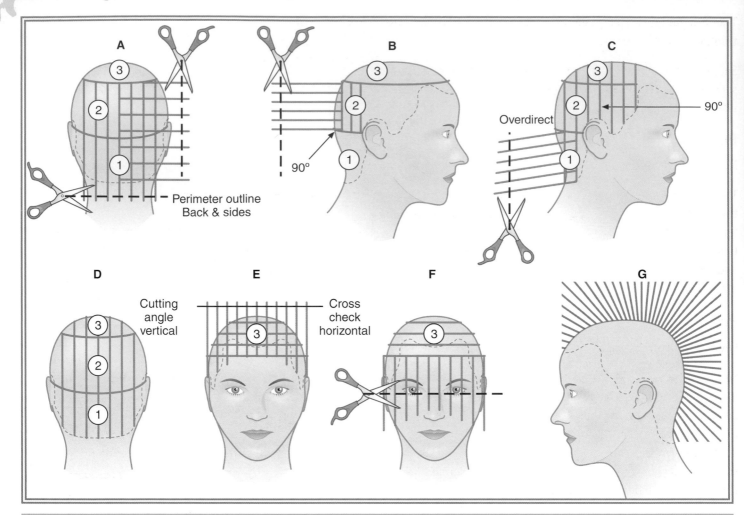

Figure 14.10 Square layers

The next perimeter hairline, section and guideline

Point 1 Sectioning

Ensure the head is in the correct position.

Point 2

Centre parting. From the centre of the forehead to the nape of the neck. Use nice clean partings to section the head into three levels.

- Level 1 Occipital bone to the ear.
- Level 2 Underneath the crown to the occipital bone. Level 2 subdivision. Repeat on the other side.
- Level 3 From underneath the crown to the frontal area.

The perimeter outline is the first guideline. Section the hair from level one starting at the nape of the neck (see Figure 14.10C).

Cutting level 1 with the perimeter outline make sure the body position is correct and that the feet are both on the floor and the client is not lopsided. Take small sections and work your way from the neck, combing downwards with the hair in its natural fall. Cut the hair as near to the skin as possible. Use a guideline.

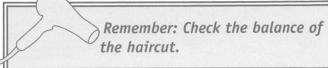

Take a little bit of the guideline for the next side. Follow this through to the other side.

Section from level 2 to behind the ear and continue to section and cut as for level 1. Repeat this for the other side.

Remember: Check the balance of the haircut.

Point 3

Now work the side section level 2.

Take horizontal sections and comb the hair down into its natural fall and cut between your fingers remembering to have the head in the correct position. When cutting around the ears release the tension through the fingers to allow the ear to take the hair up naturally. To release the tension, just open and close the fingers. Repeat this cutting technique on the other side.

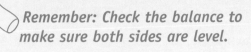

Remember: Check the balance to make sure both sides are level.

Point 4

Level 2 layering from the back section.

Section down through the middle vertically pulling the hair out at 90 degrees. Cut parallel to the section and in a straight line. Continue the back sections holding the hair out at 90 degrees travelling guideline. From just behind the ear slightly over direct to the centre to build up the length into the corners. Comb the hair underneath and on the top. Make sure that the tension is even, following the guideline through. Always follow the guideline. Cut the other side using the guide from the centre. Move the hair freely between the fingers to allow for the natural fall.

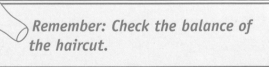

Remember: Check the balance of the haircut.

Double check that the weight of the hair is even by pulling it out at the sides between the fingers and by pulling it out towards the back.

Point 5

Side section level 2

Take vertical sections down, comb the hair out and slightly over direct back leaving the length in the perimeter and cut in a straight line. Comb the hair out at 90 degrees and cut a straight line. Cut the front of the side section last. Repeat on the other side.

Remember: Check the balance of the haircut.

Pull the hair out from the sides to check the balance and pull it from either side and pull out towards the back and centre to make sure the lengths are even.

Point 6

Level 3 from the crown to the front.

Take subsections horizontal from level 2 left side to level 2 on the right side across the crown area (see Figure 14.10). Then take a middle parting from the crown to the middle of the forehead. Comb the hair up at 90 degrees. Find the guideline from level 2. Over direct the hair and cut a straight line parallel to the section. Continue to take sections from level 2 left side to level 2 right side, pulling the hair up at 90 degrees in the middle and over directing the corners.

Start to over direct back to make the fringe longer and allow for the shape of the head being concave. Pull the sections back to ensure the fringe is longer. Cross check vertically. Check the balance through the fingers.

Point 7

Blow dry the hair using a styling lotion to finish off the cut. We use the styling lotion from the root to the end using large sections to give the hair lift and body. Make sure the product is applied evenly. If the hair is fine use mousse. Products should be used according to manufacturer's instructions.

Rounded layers

Rounded layers are also known as French crop, crop, short layers and layered haircut.

A rounded layer is a basic layer cut that can be carried out on long, short or medium length hair. The hair is pulled out at 90 degrees using a travelling guideline and cut the same length all the way round, thus giving rounded layers.

Try to use a guideline, e.g. 10 cm cut at each section. Some combs have marks to represent inches. Visual checks using mirrors and standing away from the haircut at intervals will enable you to ensure the haircut is balanced and the weight distribution even.

Again, use small sections. Always make sure you can see your guideline. If you lose your guideline, stop and go back until you can find it. Make sure each section is held out at 90 degrees. Do not under or over direct the hair.

Observe the growth patterns and head contours, as they change as you work through each step. You may need to allow for awkward hairlines and growth patterns.

Ears protrude so be careful not to catch them when combing, and always release the tension to allow the hair to fall naturally.

Techniques used to cut the rounded layer

Technique	Preparation	Reason	Look
Rounded layer on short hair. Cut on wet or dry hair (preferably wet)			Classic, fashionable, historic. More finished, can be softer if required
Cut on wet hair	Prepare by wetting the hair down	Makes the hair more manageable	
Decide on the length to be cut, e.g. 10 cm. Check the outline shape at 10 cm. Section the hair into manageable sections	Section the hair using sectioning clips. Use a cutting comb (preferably with wide teeth so as not to use too much tension) Use products if desired	To ensure the cutting section is controllable To control the hair without using too much tension Products control the hair	
	1 Section hair as in Figure 14.10a		
	2 The section line should reflect the cutting line, e.g. round following the contour of the head		
	3 Comb the hair out at 90 degrees. Cut the desired length	Ensure the cutting line follows the contour of the head	
	4 Take the next radial vertical section as shown in Figure 14.10a on level 2 directly underneath the first section 5 Use part of the previously cut section as a guideline 6 Again, comb out at 90 degrees and cut	Always take some of the previous section as a guideline	
	7 Take the next radial vertical section as shown in Figure 14.10b on level 1 directly underneath the second section. 8 Use part of the previously cut section as a guideline 9 Again comb out at 90 degrees and cut	Always take some of the previous section as a guideline	
	10 Take the next radial vertical section at level 3 next to the first section, cut as shown in Figure 14.10b on level 3 11 Use part of the previously cut section as a guideline 12 Again comb out at 90 degrees and cut	Always take some of the previous section as a guideline	

Technique	Preparation	Reason	Look
	13 Take the next radial vertical section on level 2 then level 1 and so on. Repeat this all around the head 14 Use part of the previously cut section as a guideline 15 Again comb out at 90 degrees and cut	Always take some of the previous section as a guideline	
	16 Continue taking radial vertical sections like orange segments to allow for the contours of the head 17 Use part of the previously cut section as a guideline 18 Again comb out at 90 degrees and cut 19 All sections should be 10 cm in length 20 Complete the cut by cross checking using horizontal sections	Always take some of the previous section as a guideline	
	21 Comb the perimeter outline down into its natural fall 22 Personalise the haircut to the desired length by point cutting or club cutting	The hair will be longer at the back and slightly shorter at the front as all the hair was cut to 10 cm. Therefore the perimeter will be 10 cm around the hairline	

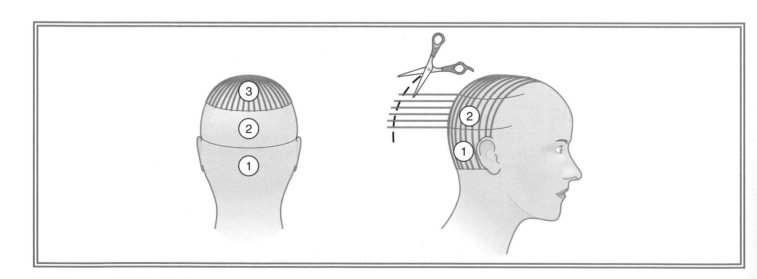

Figure 14.10a Rounded layers

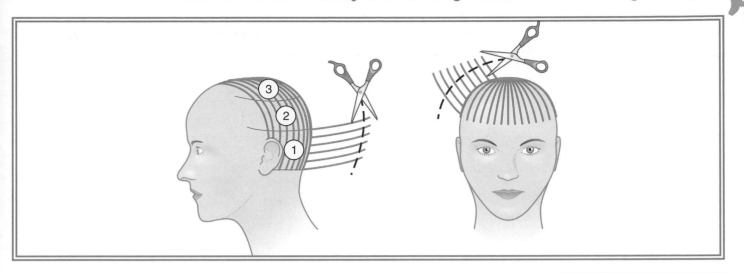

Figure 14.10b Rounded layers

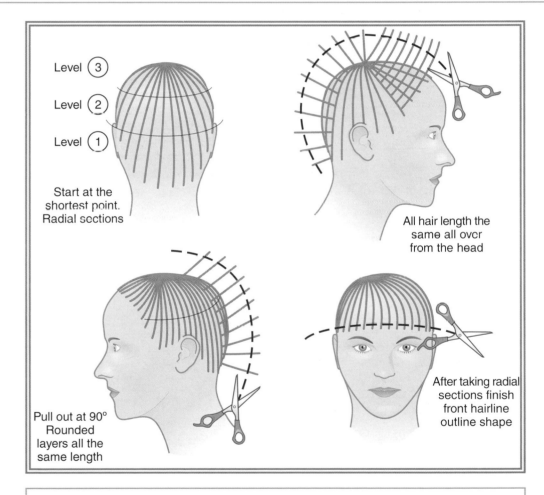

Level ③

Level ②

Level ①

Start at the shortest point. Radial sections

All hair length the same all over from the head

Pull out at 90° Rounded layers all the same length

After taking radial sections finish front hairline outline shape

Figure 14.10c Rounded layers

Graduated layers

A graduated bob is a haircut that is shorter underneath, gradually building up to longer layers on the top. It can be solid in form. Graduation bobs usually start at the nape, building up weight to the occipital bone to accentuate the shape of the head.

Use guidelines, especially as you work your way around to the front, e.g. bottom of the ear lobe. Visual checks using mirrors and standing away from the haircut at intervals will enable you to ensure the haircut is balanced and the weight distribution is even.

Again, use small sections. Always make sure you can see your guideline. If you lose your guideline, stop and go back until you can find it.

Make sure each section is held out at least 45 degrees depending on the amount of graduation required.

Observe the growth patterns and head contours as they change as you work through each step. You may need to allow for awkward hairlines and growth patterns.

Ears protrude – be careful not to catch them when combing, and always release the tension to allow the hair to fall naturally.

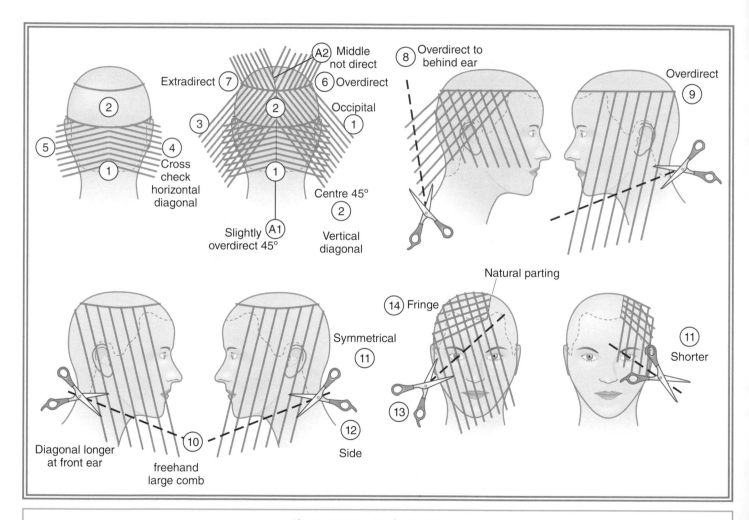

Figure 14.11 Graduated layers

Techniques used to cut the graduation bob

Technique	Preparation	Reason	Look
Graduation bob on short hair. Cut on wet or dry hair (preferably wet)			Classic, fashionable, historic. More finished, can be softer if required
Cut on wet hair	Prepare by wetting the hair down.	Makes the hair more manageable	
Decide on the length to be cut. Check the nape hairline for the outline shape. Section the hair into manageable sections	Section the hair using sectioning clips. Use a cutting comb (preferably with wide teeth so as not to use too much tension). Use products if desired	To ensure the cutting section is controllable To control the hair without using too much tension Products control the hair	
	1 Section hair as in Figure 14.11		
	2 The section line should reflect the cutting line. 3 Pull out the first section vertical and cut at 45 degrees to the head	The first section determines the height of the graduation	
	4 Now take the next section that is diagonal pointing from the centre slightly towards the ear and slightly over directing the hair to the centre 5 Cut using the guideline at 45 degrees 6 Continue these sections as in Figure 14.11 to just behind the ear 7 Repeat on the other side remembering to over direct slightly towards the centre of the head 8 Complete level 1 and cross check weight distribution 9 Take the same sections as in level 1. Use part of the previously cut section as a guideline 10 This time drop the weight down from the centre to ensure the length sits on the occipital bone and is not too high. 11 Continue working around to the side this time.	The cutting line replicates the section line Always take some of the previous section as a guideline	

Technique	Preparation	Reason	Look
	12 Continue using diagonal sections and over directing back to the centre of the head 13 Use part of the previously cut section as a guideline 14 Again comb at 45 degrees	This will make the hair increase in weight, gradually getting longer working towards the ear	

Review

The following cuts have been discussed one at a time:

- One-length bob
- Long one length square and rounded
- Square layers
- Rounded layers
- Graduated layers.

Also discussed were:

- sectioning
- hand position
- body position
- cutting lines and angles
- outline shapes
- static and travelling guidelines
- guidelines
- directing and over directing
- checking and cross checking.

There are also different cutting techniques including:

- club cutting
- razor cutting
- texturising
- slide cutting
- point cutting
- thinning
- personalising.

Haircutting shapes

There are various shapes that can be cut into the hair using either taper or club cutting:

- solid form
- uniform layering

- low layering
- reverse graduation
- increased layering.

Solid form

Most commonly known as a bob, where all the hair is cut to the same base line. This gives a 'chunky' effect to the ends of the hair and produces a square shape. There is no graduation in this hair shape and it is very useful for making finer hair appear as thick and dense as possible.

Uniform layering

The inner hair length is the same as the outer hair length. This is achieved by lifting the hair out from the head at a 90 degree angle and cutting to the same length all over, e.g. the same length at the front, sides, nape, crown, etc. This results in a round effect, which mirrors the shape of the head.

Low layering

A haircut with the inner hair length longer than the outline hair length. Pulling the hair down at a 45 degree angle, as opposed to lifting it up, creates less graduation. It is interesting to note that the less graduation there is in the hair the more of the hair bulk remains. Thus, finer hair can retain as much thickness as possible by club cutting the hair into a style with very little graduation, while thicker hair can have some of the weight or thickness removed by thinning and cutting the hair into a style that requires layering. The wedge is an example of this hair shape and the low graduation of this cut creates a triangular shape.

Reverse graduation

This technique is used when the top layers or inner length of the hair are longer than the underneath layers of the hair, e.g. a 'Bob' or 'Halo' style. In this case the inner hair length is also longer than the baseline.

Increased layering

The inner hair length is shorter than the outer hair length. Increased layering on long hair is a good example of extreme angles, where the hair is cut from short on the top or front, to long at the nape. The difference in lengths at these two points is significant and therefore the angle of the haircut is very steep. By cutting a guideline at the shortest point, then combing all the hair up to this guideline and cutting straight across at this point, very steep graduation is achieved. To cut the hair vertically and to hold the fingers at this steep angle would be very difficult and it is unlikely that each section or mesh of hair could be cut at exactly the same angle all round the head.

What is graduation?

Graduation is sometimes referred to as layering. Increased layering is when the hair is steeply graduated and low layering is when there is little graduation. Graduation can be achieved by either club cutting or taper cutting, whichever is the most suitable for the hair type and the finished dressing. It is attained when the top layers of the hair lie above the lower layers, in which case there would be a high degree of graduation, but if all the top layers lie just above the lower layers then there is less graduation.

Increasing graduation

By increasing the graduation the amount of layering in the hair is also increased. The more the hair sections are lifted, the greater the graduation. When the hair is held down close to the head, at a 0 degree angle, a bob effect is the result, which contains no graduation. At each degree of lift of hair away from the head the more graduation is achieved. To help with the understanding of the degrees of lift, it is useful to remember that a 90 degree lift means that the hair is held straight out from the head at right angles. Thus, a 45 degree lift is half this amount and a 180 degree lift is twice the lift of 90 degree.

- 45 degree lift. This will create slight graduation and is usually used for wedges, etc.
- 90 degree lift. This will create twice as much graduation and is usually used for short, uniform layered shapes.
- 180 degree lift. This will create a great deal of graduation and is usually used for long, high-layered styles.

Block graduation

Cutting a block section of hair to eliminate weight by pulling the hair upwards and out at the same level of graduation.

Curvature, concave

A rounded end shape, e.g. used on a baseline longer in the nape and shorter at the sides.

Convex

Shorter at the nape and longer at the sides. This can also be used on fringes.

Bevelling

Rounding the edges to soften the hair. Cut when hair has been built up to a point.

Natural inversion

Working a centre area of layering through the centre of the head and pulling all the rest of the hair to this point.

Pointing

Pointing the scissors into the haircut to texturise and remove hair.

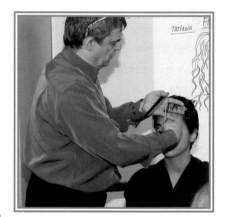

Figure 14.12 Pointing

Brick cutting

Cutting shorter pieces of hair in a brickwork fashion into existing layering. Short hair supports longer hair for body or to give texture or remove bulk.

Slicing

Sliding the scissors or razor along the hair, eliminating weight-retaining length to give texture and feather the ends.

Personalising

Designing the haircut using finishing techniques to suit the client.

Scissors over comb

This technique can cut the hair extremely short and was originally used in men's haircutting and the ladies' shingle of the 1920s. A fine, pliable comb is used to allow the hair to be cut as close to the scalp as possible. The hair is combed upwards from the nape and the hair that protrudes through the teeth of the comb is cut off. The scissors should rest along the length of the comb and should open and close quickly whilst the comb is moving up the head. If the scissors movement is too slow then steps will occur in the haircut. The angle at which the comb is held will determine the length of the hair. If it is held next to the scalp then the hair will be very short; the further away from the scalp it is held, the longer the hair. Electric or hand clippers can be used in place of the scissors and comb. The clipper heads have attachments, which

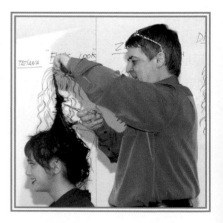

Figure 14.13 Slicing

are numbered according to their depth. Thus the lower the number the shorter it will cut the hair. A special comb known as a Brian Drummer Flat Topper can also be used with the clippers in place of the attachments. It has a spirit level incorporated into it so that the stylist can make sure that the hair is completely level when cutting.

- Baseline is the lowest point and foundation of a haircut.

- Double baseline is an additional baseline over a shorter area to create a two-dimensional effect.

- Perimeter line is the outline of a haircut.

- Internal shape is the inside area of the perimeter.

- Recession area is the front hairline where the hair recedes.

- Undercutting is cutting the underneath hair much shorter than the rest of the haircut.

- Disconnecting is leaving longer pieces of hair to accentuate the line of the haircut.

- Symmetrical means hair is the same length both sides and balanced.

- Asymmetrical means hair is longer one side than the other.

Points to remember

No matter what type of haircut is being carried out it is very important to keep the client's head in the correct position. If it is inadvertently held to one side during cutting then the finished haircut will be lopsided!

It is also important for the hair cutter to stand in the correct position, directly opposite the section of hair taken, to enable the hair to be cut evenly and squarely.

Assessing the head for cutting

It cannot be stressed too often that before placing a pair of scissors near to a head of hair, the hairdresser must know exactly what the client requires and how best to achieve that result. It is too late when the hair has been cut to realise that the client's requirements have been misunderstood, or even ignored! Clients are often nervous when they visit a salon for the first time, particularly when they require a haircut. Talking to the client and discussing the requirements enables the hairdresser to find out exactly what the client needs and expects from the haircut. It also helps to build up a relationship of trust and confidence between the client and the hairdresser.

To prevent unnecessary mishaps, and to gain enough information to allow the hairdresser to proceed with confidence, two main areas must be explored:

- assessment of the client.

- assessment of the hair.

Assessment of the client

This is meant to determine the client's requirements and enables the hairdresser to advise the client on any modifications of the chosen haircut that may be necessary. It is important to question the client closely: they may know exactly what they have in mind but have great difficulty in describing the exact haircut. If this is the case, it is often useful to keep a book of fashionable hairstyles available in the salon to show the client. Thus, the hairdresser will have a visual description of the style or look that the client is aiming for.

The following factors must also be taken into consideration, as they will influence the suitability of the chosen haircut:

- face shape and prominent features

- neck length

- body size

- age, hobbies and lifestyle.

Face shape and prominent features

The finished shape of the haircut should suit and flatter the client. This seems a very obvious statement, but it is surprising how many hairdressers disregard the shape of the client's face when restyling the hair. Take a good look at the client's face by drawing the hair away from the face to determine whether it is round, square, long, oval, etc. This can affect the amount of hair that needs to be removed and will also help to determine the shape of the finished haircut. Next, check whether there are any prominent features or blemishes that need to be camouflaged, e.g. a receding chin. Some prominent features can be attractive and therefore need to be emphasised, e.g. the eyes can be emphasised by a fringe.

Neck length

If the client has a very long neck the hair needs to be left longer in the nape. Alternatively, a very short neck looks less obvious if the hair is kept shorter in the nape or is swept up towards the top of the head to make the neck appear longer.

Body size

The finished haircut should be part of a total look, not just a separate item that happens to be attached to the client's head! For example, a very tall, slim client with a small head would look ridiculous with a short, scalp-hugging haircut.

Age, hobbies and lifestyle

The age of the client is a very important consideration. A middle-aged person does not always suit the same style as a teenager, although a current fashion trend can often be adapted to meet the needs of both, as long as it is not too extreme. The general lifestyle and hobbies of the client also need to be considered. When assessing a client's personality, clothes, etc, it is important not to gown up until you are starting the procedure. Also find out if the client will have enough spare time to spend on an elaborate hairstyle or whether they will need a style that requires the minimum amount of time spent on it between salon visits. These and many other questions need to be asked to find out exactly what the client expects and requires of the haircut.

Assessment of the hair

This is to determine the type and method of cutting to use. Remember that it is sometimes necessary to combine a variety of haircutting techniques on one head to achieve the required shape. Whenever possible, use the type of hair to its best advantage – it is very difficult, if not impossible, to create a long, smooth bob style on very thick, naturally curly hair. It is far better to utilise the curl and thickness of the hair to create a style that requires these features. Consider the following:

- hair texture
- hair volume
- hair length
- amount of natural curl or movement present in the hair
- growth direction of the hair.

Hair texture

The texture of the hair refers to the diameter of the hair and can either be fine, thick or medium. Fine hair will need all the bulk retained; heavy club cutting helps to do this. Thick or coarse hair may need to have some of the bulk removed, in which case it may be necessary to thin, taper or high layer the hair, depending upon the finished style. Medium textured hair is usually no problem and adapts to most cutting techniques, again depending upon the finished style.

Hair volume

This is the amount of hair on the scalp, or how densely the hair grows. A client may have fine textured hair, but with plenty of hairs on the scalp making it quite abundant or they may have thick, coarse hair, which is very sparse. The density of hair can vary throughout the head, e.g. hair may be denser at the nape than the crown. Therefore, there are many combinations making each head slightly different.

Hair length

Clients do not always realise that some haircuts require a lot of length in certain areas and often do not appreciate how long it takes for the hair to grow to the length they require. Often it is necessary to compromise with a hairstyle, and it may take a few months and quite a few haircuts to achieve the final effect. A good example of this is when a client has had a layered or steeply graduated haircut and wishes to grow out the top layers until the hair is all one length. This can take up to twelve months, depending upon how short the hair was originally.

Advice should be given to the client on the type of styles and haircuts they can have during this period, in order to keep the hair well shaped without loss of length from the areas that need to grow longer.

Amount of natural curl or movement present in the hair

Always try to use any natural curl or movement in the hair. Ignoring or fighting against the curl can often ruin a haircut. By using and incorporating any natural curl or movement the haircut will stay in shape longer and will be easier for the client to manage.

Growth direction of the hair

Strong growth direction patterns can cause some difficulties when cutting the hair, e.g. a double crown, strong nape line, etc. Cutting the hair when wet without tension allows extra length in these areas and prevents an uneven line when the haircut is finished.

Sections for cutting

Sections are necessary when cutting hair to allow the hairdresser to proceed with the haircut in a neat and methodical manner. When cutting a basic haircut it is often more efficient to commence cutting at the nape. Sectioning is necessary therefore to hold the remaining hair firmly out of the way for greater ease when working.

Cutting angles around the hairline

The hair may be cut at many angles around the hairline to create different shapes and styles. Always remember to take into consideration any strong hair growth direction patterns, e.g. strong nape line, cows-lick, etc.

Cross checking the line

After cutting any head of hair the haircut should be checked very thoroughly across the sections to ensure that it is level and even from all angles. This is known as cross–checking. However, remember when cross-checking a fashion cut not to get too enthusiastic and alter the line or shape of the style, particularly if the angles already cut are very steep. Check carefully around the hairline at the sides, front and nape. If the hair has been held and cut away from the head, the underneath hair will be slightly longer, leaving wisps of hair that can make the finished line untidy. Unless this was intended to be part of the finished style they should be removed.

Basic guidelines when cutting hair

1 Decide the exact shape of the finished haircut before starting to cut the hair.

2 Choose the correct type of cutting necessary for the type of hair.

3 Always cut a guideline from which to work.

4 Cut the guideline at the shortest point of the haircut.

5 Comb each section of hair to be cut cleanly and thoroughly from the root to the point.

6 Do not take cutting sections that are too large. The guideline must be clearly visible through the mesh.

7 Try to cut the hair on a straight line as this gives a more precise result. Use the fact that the head is a round object to create the angles, rather than holding the hair, scissors or fingers at an awkward angle.

8 Cut with the hair growth direction and utilise any natural curl or movement to enhance the style.

9 Never cut the hair too short. It is easy to remove more hair but impossible to put it back on again.

10 When cutting wet hair allow for the fact that hair will lift 5 mm (¼") when dry.

11 When precision cutting, do not allow the hair to dry out. Always keep it evenly wet.

12 When cutting around the ear, allow for ear protrusion and do not cut the hair too short.

13 Always cross-check a basic haircut by lifting the hair away from the head in the opposite direction from which it has been cut.

14 Give a final check to the haircut when the hair is dry and dressed.

15 Always advise the client on the care and maintenance of their haircut, especially if they have had a new style.

16 For beginners – if the guideline at the nape is cut with the client's head bent forward it will help to avoid the risk of cutting the hairline too short when the head is lifted upright.

17 Be aware of the health and safety of the client and yourself at all times.

18 Dispose of sharps safely (see health and safety, Unit G1 and Unit G9).

19 Sterilise tools (see health and safety, Unit G1 and Unit G9).

20 Maintain electrical equipment, e.g. keep in safe working order, no trailing flexes, disconnect after use, make sure hands are dry before switching on, oil clippers regularly, etc.

21 Choose the correct type of cutting tools necessary for the type of haircut. Ensure they are sharp and rust free. Maintain them by keeping them sharpened or using new blades for razor cuts, etc. Clipper heads should be balanced and renewed or checked as needed. Ensure combs and clips are of a professional standard and not broken, etc. Always sterilise after use.

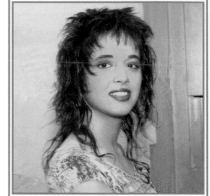

Figure 14.14

Combination haircuts

Combination cutting techniques will help you to plan and execute the right haircut to balance the client's head shape if done correctly. Combination haircuts are those where you use more than one technique to create a variety of looks, e.g. one length technique, followed by forward graduation then personalised using slide cutting and texturising techniques giving you more control.

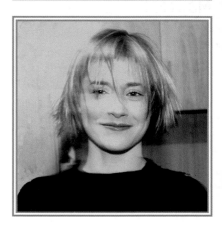

Figure 14.15

Remember the consultation to ensure you have agreed to exactly what the client requires (read through Unit G9). With this service you need to pay particular attention to the following:

- Client's personal details, age, growth patterns, hair type, shape of head and body, density, texture, condition, distinguishing marks, features, contraindications, and hair length, etc.

- How often does the client visit the hair salon? How do they style their hair? What products do they use?

- Is there anything they do not like about their hair? What has worked well for them in the past? Is the haircut realistic in terms of length and texture, etc?

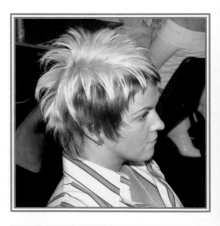

Figure 14.16

It is all about getting the balance right and distributing weight to complement the head shape. Look at the shape of the head carefully. Some clients have small heads and therefore more length may be needed to balance this. Some clients' occipital bone is very flat and therefore more weight may be needed to compensate. No two head shapes are the same and together with the facial features and different hair types, each client's needs are different.

Additional information
Useful websites

Website Addresses	Content
www.habia.org.uk	Hairdressing and Beauty Industry Authority. Downloads available including references to other websites
www.lookfantastic.com	Professional hairdressing products and advice
www.laurandp.co.uk	Educational publications for development of professional hairdressing
www.scott999.fsnet.co.uk	Hairdressing product information
www.nexus.com	Range of hairdressing products
www.tigi.co.uk	Range of hairdressing products, cutting videos
www.vidalsassoon.co.uk	Range of hairdressing products, cutting videos

Magazines and journals

- *Hairdressers Journal*
- *Creative Head*
- *Estetica/Cutting Edge*
- *Black Beauty and Hair*

ACTIVITY

Outcome 1

- *Describe the correct use of cutting equipment and the effects they have on the hair.*
- *Explain how to maintain cutting equipment.*
- *Describe the effects created by different haircutting techniques and effects; graduating, club cutting, layering, scissor over comb, clipper over comb, texturising, razoring, freehand, tapering and thinning.*
- *State why factors, including client requirements, hair texture, growth patterns, head/face shapes/features, need to be considered when cutting hair.*
- *Explain safety considerations that must be taken into account when cutting hair.*
- *Describe the range of current fashion looks for women, men, teenagers and children.*
- *State the importance of applying tension when cutting hair.*
- *State the factors that need to be considered when cutting wet and dry hair.*
- *Explain how to dispose of sharps safely.*
- *Explain how to check and look after electrical equipment for safe use.*

15 UNIT H28 PROVIDE COLOUR CORRECTION SERVICES

1 Maintain effective and safe methods of working when correcting hair colour

2 Determine the problem

3 Plan and agree a course of action to correct colour

4 Correct colour

CHAPTER CONTENTS

- *Colour Correction*
- *Re-colouring Following Colour Correction*
- *Precautions*
- *Hair Structure and Pigmentation*
- *Types of Hair Colour*

It is recommended that you read Chapter 17 to recap on types of colour etc.

Colour correction

An unwanted discoloration of the hair can usually be corrected by the addition of another colour. Look at the two triangles that form 'The Colour Circle'.

- One with **the primary colours**.
- One with **the secondary colours**.
- Orange discoloration is corrected by its opposite colour – blue.
- Yellow discoloration is corrected by its opposite colour – purple.
- Green discoloration is corrected by its opposite colour – red.
- Red discoloration is corrected by its opposite colour – green.

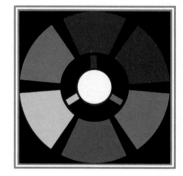

Figure 15.1 The colour circle

When masking unwanted colour the depth is very important, e.g. pale yellow can be corrected by using pale purple. In other words, hair that has been bleached or highlighted and appears yellow can be toned down by using toners containing pale purple pigment to produce a beige blonde.

The colour problem

Your colour result hasn't turned out quite as expected. The colour has developed two depths too dark and the tone is much too copper for your client's liking.

Your normal colour correction solution . . .

- Counteract the copper with an ash-based tone, knowing that the depth will still remain the same?
- Prepare a bleach bath to strip the depth and tone from the hair?

There are various products on the market that will help you to remove unwanted permanent colour. When removing colour you need to ensure you leave the hair in good condition. All hairdressers should have a product available for removing colour just in case something goes wrong. No matter how careful you are problems can occur so it is always good to have a contingency plan in place.

Before you use any of these products always read the manufacturer's instructions as they can vary. Carry out a consultation and all necessary tests before applying the product to the client's hair. Make sure you use the right product for the job. Carry out an incompatibility test to make sure it is permanent colour you are dealing with and not henna compounds or metallic dyes. Carry out a skin test. See Chapter 1 for more information.

Re-colouring following colour correction

At the end of either reduction process, the hair is now ready to be re-coloured. Immediately after reduction the hair will accept colour more easily.

When re-colouring the hair it is advisable to choose a shade that is one level lighter than the target shade (using the appropriate developer). In cases where copper and violet tones are used, 9% (30 vol) developer is recommended.

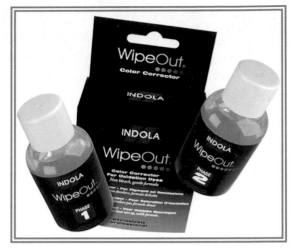

Figure 15.2 One of the colour correction products available

Remember: Semi-dry the hair before re-colouring.

To ensure the hair does not become too dark, frequently check the development of the shade you have chosen.

Precautions

- Strand test recommended prior to colouring.
- Always wear gloves.
- Protect clothing during application.
- Avoid contact with eyes. Rinse immediately if product comes into contact with them.

There are many exciting ranges of colour available that offer you all that you may need to create your desired effect. Some are specifically designed to encourage the ultimate colour creativity.

Hair structure and pigmentation

Hair is made of keratin, a complex protein containing sulphur, carbon, hydrogen, nitrogen and oxygen. The sulphur determines the strength of the hair because these chemical links are the most difficult to break down. Like all proteins, keratin comprises chains of amino acids of which there are 23 known types; 17 of these can be found in hair.

Melanin colours the hair black or brown. Pheomelanin colours it red or yellow. The colour you see therefore depends on the amounts and proportions of these pigments. Granules of pigment then form in different shapes and sizes. Generally the larger colour pigments are black, brown and red in colour. The smaller ones are orange, yellow and pale yellow colours.

All natural hair colour is a mixture of black, brown, red, orange and yellow pigments. The amount and density of each of these determines the overall colour. Grey hair is a mix of colourless and natural coloured hair and is not always due to ageing. It could be as a result of a number of factors including ill-health, shock or a lack of vitamins. 'Greyness' is often expressed as a percentage of white hair. For example '50% white' means that half the hairs on the head are white and half are their original colour.

- Black and dark brown hair is 40% black/30% brown/20% red/10% yellow
- Light brown hair is 20% black/25% brown/25% red/30% yellow
- Blonde hair is 5% black/10% brown/20% red/65% yellow

Types of hair colour

Permanent colour

Permanent colour changes the natural colour of hair. When tiny colour molecules are mixed with hydrogen peroxide the colour penetrates the cuticle and is absorbed into the cortex. Oxidation takes place causing the molecules to expand so the new colour remains permanently fixed within the hair. Permanent colours can lighten and colour, or darken and colour, natural hair in one application. The most usual forms of this type of colour are cream, gel or liquid.

Bleaching

Bleach is a substance used to lift colour from the hair. Once combined with hydrogen peroxide, the mixture causes the hair to swell and raise the cuticle to allow the bleach to penetrate into the cortex. Oxidation takes place and the natural colour pigments are gradually removed (changed into a colourless compound) in the following order: black – brown – red – orange – yellow.

UNIT H29 PERM HAIR USING A VARIETY OF TECHNIQUES

1 Maintain effective and safe methods of working when perming hair

2 Prepare for perming

3 Create a variety of permed effects

CHAPTER CONTENTS

- History of Permanent Waving
- Hair Structure and Perming
- Perming Techniques
- Perm preparation
- Alternative Perming Techniques

- Preliminary (Pre-perm) Test Curls
- Problems and Solutions
- Important safety precautions
- Additional Information
- Activity

Introduction

Chemical processes including permanent waving enable you, the hairdresser, to offer a wide range of hairstyles and effects to your clients. This in turn enables you to satisfy your client's needs and is most lucrative financially.

The wide variety of products and the range of techniques available enable you to produce many differing effects, from those that show little obvious effect but support the style to those that have a dramatic, obvious effect. The properly completed perm provides many valuable benefits to both your client and you the stylist:

- long-lasting style retention
- easy manageability for your client when styling at home
- additional volume and fullness for styling soft, fine hair textures
- greater control in styling hair that is naturally coarse, wiry and hard to manage.

These processes must be carried out with due care, as the chemicals used when permanently curling hair, if used incorrectly, may cause damage to the hair and even injury to your client. Always follow the manufacturer's directions for safe use.

History of permanent waving

Attempts to wave and curl straight hair date back to early civilisation. Egyptian and Roman women were known to apply a mixture of soil and water to their hair, wrap it on crudely made wooden rollers, and then bake it in the sun. The results, of course, were not always permanent.

The machine age of permanent waving

In 1905 Charles Nessler invented a heavily wired machine that supplied electrical current to metal rods around which hair strands were wrapped. These heavy units were heated during the perming process. They were kept from touching the scalp by a complex system of counterbalancing weights, suspended from an overhead chandelier mounted on a stand (see Figure 16.1).

Two methods were used to wind hair strands around the metal units. Long hair was wound from the scalp to the ends, a technique called spiral winding (see Figure 16.2). After World War I, when many women cut their hair into the short bobbed style, the croquignole winding technique was introduced (see Figure 16.3). Using this method, shorter hair was wound from the ends towards the scalp. The hair was then styled into deep waves with loose end curls.

The client's fear of being 'tied' to an electrical contraption with the possibility of receiving a shock or burn led to the development of alternative methods of waving hair. In 1931, the pre-heat method of perming was introduced. Hair was wrapped using the croquignole method, and then clamps, pre-heated by a separate electrical unit, were placed over the wound curls. This was known as the falling heat or wireless system.

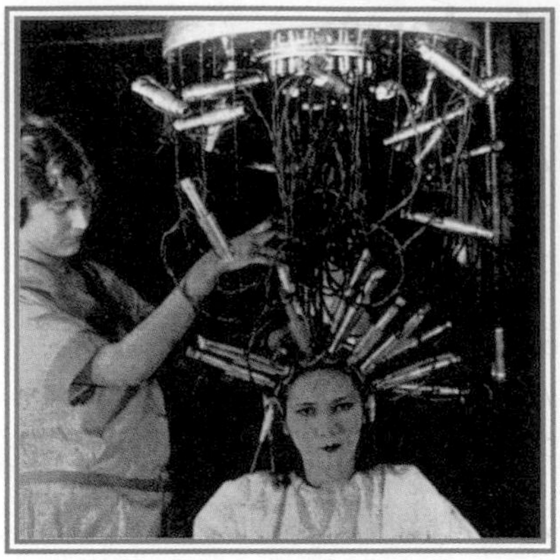

Figure 16.1 Machine permanent wave

The first machineless perm

An alternative to the machine perm was introduced in 1932 when chemists Ralph L. Evans and Everett G. McDonough pioneered a method that used external heat generated by chemical reaction. Small, flexible pads, called exothermic pads, containing a chemical mixture, calcium oxide, were wound around hair strands. When the pads were moistened with water, a chemical heat was released that created long-lasting curls. Thus the first machineless permanent wave was born. Salon clients were no longer subjected to the dangers and discomforts of the Nessler machine.

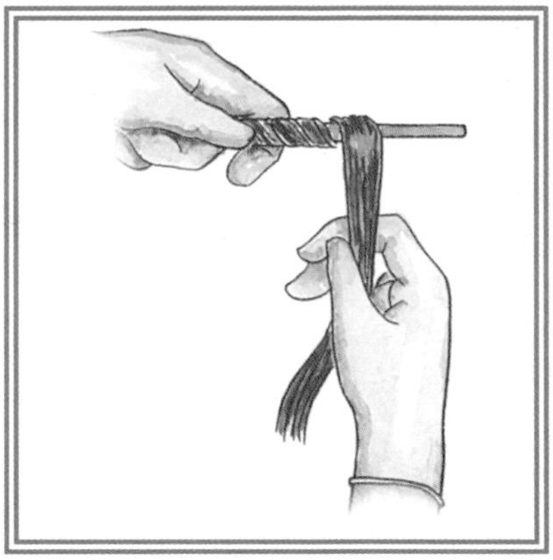

Figure 16.2 Spiral flat wind

Cold waves

In 1941 scientists discovered another method of permanent waving. They developed the waving lotion, a liquid that softens and expands the hair strand. After the waving lotion has done its work, another lotion called a neutraliser is applied. The neutraliser hardens and shrinks that hair strand, allowing it to conform to the shape of the rod around which the hair is wrapped. It also stops the action of the waving lotion.

Because this perm does not use heat, it is called a 'cold wave'. Cold waves replaced virtually all predecessors and competitors, and cold waving and permanent waving became almost synonymous terms. Modern versions of cold waves, usually referred to as alkaline perms, are still very popular today.

Note: The word 'perm' is now popularly used to indicate permanent waving with either alkaline or acid balanced solution.

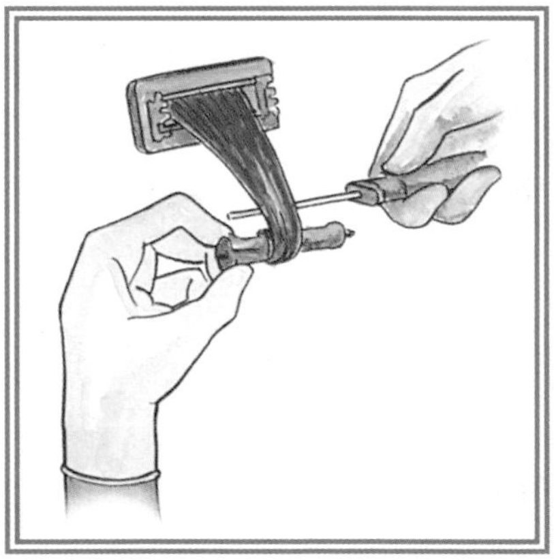

Figure 16.3 Croquignole wind

Acid-balanced perms

For many years, manufacturers sought to develop a permanent wave solution that would minimise hair damage and permit hair that had been damaged by lightening or tinting services to receive a perm. To achieve these goals, they developed a waving lotion that was not as highly alkaline as earlier lotions. Acid-balanced permanent waves with pH levels ranging from 4.5 to 7.9 were introduced in 1970. They did not contain strong alkalis and were therefore less damaging to the hair. Acid-balanced lotions were, however, slow to penetrate hair, and processing time was longer. To overcome this problem, the client is placed under a pre-heated hood dryer to shorten the processing time. Often the curl pattern achieved from acid-balanced perms is softer than that achieved from a cold wave; therefore a size smaller perm rod is often advised.

Modern perm chemistry

Perm chemistry is constantly being refined and improved. Perms are available today in many differing formulas for a wide variety of hair types. Waving lotions and neutralisers for both acid-balanced and alkaline perms are being formulated with new conditioners, proteins and natural ingredients that help to protect (buffer) and condition the hair during and after perming.

Stop-action processing is incorporated in many waving lotions to ensure optimum curl development. The curling takes place within a fixed time without the risk of over processing or damaging the hair. Special pre-wrapping lotions have also been developed to compensate for hair that is not equally porous all over.

Virtually all permanent waves are achieved with a two-step chemical process:

1 Waving lotion, which softens or breaks the internal structure of the hair.

2 Neutraliser, which re-hardens or rebonds the internal structure of the hair.

The pH scale

This 14-point scale is used to indicate the acidity or alkalinity of a substance. The symbol pH (potential Hydrogen) refers to the quantity of hydrogen ions present. The centre of the scale is neutral (7) and is a point that is neither acid or alkali. The further from the central point, the higher the level of either acidity (pH 1–7) or alkalinity (pH 7–14). Figure 3.17 indicates the relative pH of a number of hairdressing-related substances.

Care should be taken when handling any substance whose pH falls near the extremes of the scale as they may cause injury to the skin.

Alkaline perms

The main active ingredient or reducing agent in alkaline perms, ammonium thioglycolate, is a chemical compound made up of ammonium hydroxide and thioglycolic acid. The pH of alkaline waving lotions generally falls within the range of 8.2 to 9.6, depending on the amounts of ammonium hydroxide. Because the lotion is more alkaline, the cuticle layers swell slightly and open, allowing the solution to penetrate more quickly than acid-balanced lotions. Some alkaline perms are wrapped with waving lotion (pre-damping), others with water (post-damping). Some require a plastic cap (to retain scalp heat) for processing, others do not. Therefore, it is extremely important to read the manufacturer's instructions for use, before beginning.

The benefits of alkaline perms are:

- strong curl patterns
- fast processing time (varies from 5 minutes to 20 minutes)
- room temperature processing.

Generally, alkaline perms should be used when:

- perming resistant hair
- a strong/tight curl is desired
- the client has a history of early curl relaxation.

Acid-balanced perms

The main active ingredient in acid-balanced waving lotions is glycerol monothioglycolate, which effectively reduces the pH. This lower pH is gentler on the hair and typically gives a softer curl than alkaline cold waves. Acid-balanced perms have a pH range of approximately 4.5 to 7.9 and usually penetrate the hair more slowly. Thus, they require a longer processing time and heat for curl development. Heat is used in one of two ways:

1 The perm is activated by heat created chemically within the product. This method is called exothermic.

2 The perm is activated by an outside heat source, usually a conventional hood-type hair dryer. This method is called endothermic.

Recent advances in acid-balanced perm chemistry, however, have made it possible to process some acid-balanced perms at room temperature without heat. These newer acid-balanced perms usually have a slightly higher pH but still contain glycerol monothioglycolate as the active ingredient.

All acid-balanced perms are water wrapped, require a plastic cap (to retain scalp heat), and may or may not require a pre-heated hood dryer for processing. Read the manufacturer's perm directions carefully before starting the perm.

The benefits of acid-balanced perms are:

● softer curl patterns

● slower, but more controllable, processing time (usually 15 to 25 minutes)

● gentler treatment for delicate hair types.

Generally, acid-balanced perms are used when:

● perming delicate/fragile or colour-treated hair

● soft, natural curl or wave pattern is desired

● style support, rather than strong curl, is required.

The chemistry of neutralisers

Neutralisers for both acid-balanced and alkaline perms have the same important function: to establish the new curl shape permanently. Neutralising is a very important step in the perming process. If the hair is not properly neutralised, the curl will relax or straighten within one to two shampooings. Generally, today's neutralisers are composed of a relatively small percentage of hydrogen peroxide, an oxidising agent, and at an acidic pH. As with waving lotions, there are slightly different procedures recommended for individual products. To achieve the best possible results, read and follow the manufacturer's directions.

Hair structure and perming

Whether using an acid-balanced or alkaline formula, all perms subject the hair to two different actions:

1 Physical action – wrapping sections of hair around a perm rod.

2 Chemical action – created first by reducing agent (waving lotion) and second by an oxidising agent (neutraliser).

Since both of these actions work together to create a change in the internal structure of the hair, it is important to understand the composition of hair and how it is affected during perming.

Physical structure of hair

Each strand of hair is structurally subdivided into three major components:

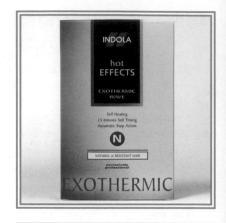

Figure 16.4 Exothermic perm

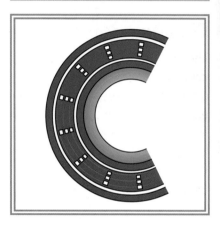

Figure 16.5 During processing, waving lotion breaks the chemical cross-bonds (links) permitting the hair to adjust to the curvature of the rod while in this softened condition

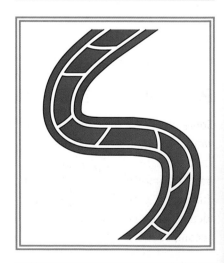

Figure 16.6 The neutraliser re-forms the chemical bonds (links) to conform with the wound position of the hair, and re-hardens the hair, thus creating the permanent wave

1. The cuticle or outer covering consists of seven or more overlapping layers. Although it comprises a small percentage of the total weight of hair, the cuticle possesses unique structural properties that protect the hair. During perming, the waving lotion raises the cuticle layers and allows the active ingredients to enter the cortex.

2. The cortex, the major component of the hair structure, accounts for up to 90% of its total weight. The cortex gives hair its flexibility, elasticity, strength, resilience and colour. It is in the cortex that the physical and chemical actions take place during the perming process to restructure the hair into a new curl configuration.

3. The medulla is the innermost section of the hair structure. The function of the medulla, if any, is unknown. In fact, it is not at all unusual for an otherwise normal, healthy hair to be without a medulla.

Chemical composition of hair

The chemical composition of hair consists almost entirely of a protein material called keratin, which is made up of approximately 19 amino acids. When many acids are bonded together, they form a polypeptide chain. These chains intertwine around each other in a spiral fashion to assume a helical shape very similar to a spring. Hair contains a high concentration of the amino acid cystine, which is joined together crosswise with disulphide linkages or bonds. Disulphide bonds add strength to the keratin protein, and it is these bonds that must be broken down to allow the perming process to occur.

Processing

The chemical action of a waving lotion breaks the disulphide bonds and softens the hair. When the chemical action softens the inner structure of the hair enough, it can mould to the shape of the rod around which it is wound (see Figure 16.7–16.9).

Neutralising

When the hair has assumed the desired shape, the broken disulphide bonds must be chemically re-bonded. Neutralising re-hardens the hair and fixes it into its new curl form. When the neutralising action is completed, the hair is unwrapped from the rods, and you have a new curl formation (see Figures 16.5 and 16.6).

Perming techniques

Some alkaline perm product directions call for water wrapping, some are lotion wrapped, and others require pre-wrap lotions. Some wave lotions come in two parts that must be mixed just prior to use. Some need dryer heat. (Note: the dryer should be pre-heated). Some perms require that a plastic cap be placed over the curlers during the processing, others do not. Considering all the variables, it is not a good idea to trust your memory. Make it a practice to check the printed directions that accompany every perm each time you give a perm.

The stages of perming:

1. Client consultation
2. Selection of equipment and products
3. Pre-perm shampooing

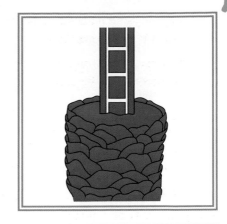

Figure 16.7 Each hair strand is composed of many polypeptide chains. This series of illustrations shows the behaviour of one such chain

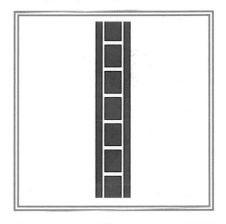

Figure 16.8 Hair before processing. Chemical bonds (links) give hair its strength and firmness

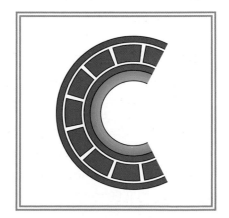

Figure 16.9 Hair wound on the rod. The hair bends to the curvature and size of the rod

4 Sectioning and parting

5 The perm wind/wrap

6 Applying waving lotion

7 Processing time

8 Testing curls during processing

9 Water rinsing

10 Neutralising/normalising

11 Post-perm precautions

How do you decide which perming technique is right for your client? You must be able to evaluate and analyse your client's hair. You must consult with your client to establish what they expect to accomplish with a perm – a tight, curly look or a loose, wavy look. This information helps you to select the correct perm product and technique.

Client consultation

Every perm client has a different expectation for how he or she wants the perm to look. The only way to meet your client's expectations is to determine what those expectations are. Talk to your client in a friendly, but professional way. Take a few minutes to discuss:

1 What hairstyle and how much curl your client wants. Photos or magazine pictures help to make this clearly understood by both of you.

2 Your client's life-style. Does he or she have leisure time, or a demanding schedule that requires a low-maintenance style?

3 How your client's hairstyle relates to overall personal image. Is your client concerned about current fashion trends?

4 Your client's previous experience with perming. What did he or she like or dislike about past perm services?

Once you learn the questions to ask and how to ask them, the consultation with your perm client will take only a few minutes. It is time well spent, however, because the consultation helps establish your credibility as a professional. It inspires your client's confidence in your technical and creative abilities, and makes the perming experience more satisfactory for both of you. See Chapter 3 for further information.

Remember: If the presence of previous, unknown chemical treatments is apparent, carry out an incompatibility test, to test for the presence of metallic salts on the hair (see Unit G1).

Keep the vital information you learn during the client consultation as a permanent record, either written or computerised, along with other important data, including the client's address, home and business phone numbers.

Perm preparation

Selection of equipment and products

Before you begin perming, make sure you have all the necessary materials at hand. Good organisation and planning will help to develop precision and speed in completing a perm. At the perming station the following equipment should be laid out in an organised, easily accessible fashion:

1 The perm product.

2 Client's record card.

3 Towels.

4 Curlers (organised by size).

5 Plastic hair clips and pins.

6 End papers.

7 Pin tail comb.

8 Cotton wool.

9 Protective gloves.

10 Perm lotion applicator.

> *Remember: Always read and follow the manufacturer's instructions carefully.*

Pre-perm analysis

After the client consultation, you must analyse the overall condition of your client's hair and scalp. This analysis is essential for you to determine:

> *Caution: If pre-perm analysis is not correct, poor curl development or hair damage can result.*

- if it is safe and advisable to proceed with the perm service. The hair must be in good condition and have the necessary strength to accept a chemical alteration to achieve a successful perm

- which perm product should be chosen for the best results on the particular hair type

- which perm technique should be used: curler/rod and parting sizes and winding/wrapping pattern.

First, examine the scalp for abrasions, irritations, open sores or contagious disorders. If any of these exist, do not give the perm. Minor abrasions may be protected by using petroleum jelly BP as a barrier between the skin and the lotion. Next, judge the physical characteristics of the hair with regard to these important criteria: porosity, density, texture, length. Finally, determine the overall condition of the hair. Observe if the hair has been previously treated with chemicals: perm, tint, bleach, highlighting (frosting, dimensionally coloured). This will guide you in choosing the appropriate perm.

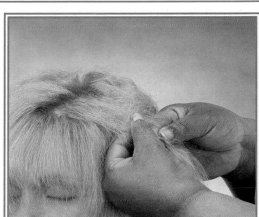

Figure 16.10 Checking for hair porosity

Determining porosity

Porosity refers to the hair's capacity to absorb moisture. There is a direct relationship between the hair's porosity, the type of perm (acid-balanced or alkaline) you will use, and the strength of waving lotion you will choose.

The processing time for any perm depends more on hair porosity than any other factor. The more porous the hair, the less processing time it takes and a milder waving solution is required. The degree to which hair absorbs the waving lotion is related to its porosity, regardless of texture.

Hair porosity is affected by such factors as excessive exposure to sun and wind, use of harsh shampoos, tints and lighteners, previous perms and use of thermal styling appliances.

Porous hair might be dry – even very dry. If hair is tinted, bleached, has been exposed to sun or was over-processed by a previous perm, it will absorb liquids readily. Soft, fine, thin hair usually has a thin cuticle so it will absorb liquids quickly and easily. Rough, dull-looking hair and hair that tangles easily are also signs of porous hair.

While the hair is dry, check porosity in three different areas: front hairline, in front of the ear and in the crown area. Select a single strand of hair, hold the end securely between the thumb and first finger of one hand and slide the thumb and first finger of the other hand from the hair end to the scalp.

If the hair feels smooth and the cuticle is dense and hard, it is considered resistant and will not absorb liquids or perm lotion easily. If you can feel a slight roughness, this tells you that the cuticle is open and that the hair is porous and will absorb liquids more readily (see Figure 16.10).

Poor porosity (resistant hair)

Hair with the cuticle layer lying close to the hair shaft. This type of hair absorbs waving lotion slowly and usually requires a longer processing time and/or a strong waving lotion.

Good porosity (normal hair)

Hair with the cuticle layer slightly raised from the hair shaft. Hair of this type can absorb moisture or chemicals in an average amount of time.

Porous (tinted, lightened or previously chemically treated) hair

Hair that has been made porous by various treatments or styling. This type of hair absorbs lotion very quickly and requires the shortest processing time. Use either an acid-balanced perm or a very mild alkaline wave.

Over-porous hair (a result of over processing)

This type of hair is very damaged, dry, fragile and brittle. Until the hair has been reconditioned or the damaged part has been removed by cutting, it should not be permed.

If hair is unevenly porous (usually porous or over porous at the ends with good to poor porosity near the scalp), a pre-wrap lotion, specifically designed to even out the porosity, is recommended to achieve even curl results and help prevent over-processing porous ends (see Figures 16.11 – 16.14).

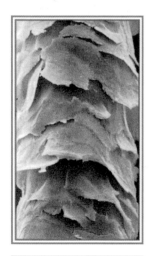
Figure 16.11 Damaged (over-porous hair)

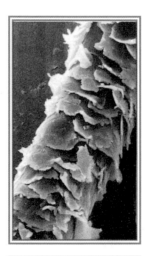
Figure 16.12 Tinted (extreme porosity

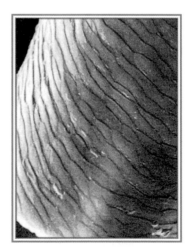
Figure 16.13 Resistant (poor porosity)

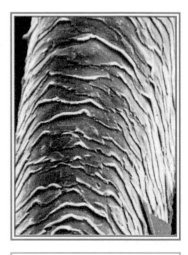
Figure 16.14 Normal (moderate porosity)

Determining texture

Texture refers to how thick or thin (in diameter) each individual hair is. Fine hair has a small diameter; coarse hair has a large diameter. You can feel whether hair is fine, coarse or medium when a single dry strand is held between the fingers.

The texture and porosity together are used to determine the processing time of the waving lotion. Although porosity is the more important of the two, texture does play an important role in estimating processing time. Fine hair with a small diameter becomes saturated with waving lotion more quickly than coarse hair with a large diameter, even if both are of equal porosity. However, when coarse hair is porous, it processes faster than fine hair that is not porous.

A perm adds body to hair that appears limp, lifeless, and does not hold a style very long. For coarse, wiry hair, a perm provides greater manageability in styling (see Figure 16.15).

Testing elasticity

Elasticity is the ability of hair to stretch and then return to its original length. To test for elasticity, stretch a single dry hair. If the hair breaks under very slight strain, it has little or no elasticity. Other signs of poor elasticity include a spongy feel when the hair is wet and/or hair that tangles easily. When hair is completely lacking in elasticity (for example, extremely damaged hair), it will not take a satisfactory permanent wave because it has lost the ability to contract after stretching. The greater the degree of elasticity, the longer the wave will remain in the hair, because less relaxation of the hair occurs. Hair with good elastic qualities can be stretched 20% of its length without breaking (see Figure 16.16).

Assessing density

Density, or thickness, refers to the number of hairs per square centimetre (0.155 sq. inch) on your client's head. Density is one characteristic that determines the size of the partings you will use. Thick hair (many hairs per square centimetre) will require small partings on each rod. Too much hair on the rod can result in a weak curl, especially at the scalp.

If hair is thin (fewer hairs per square centimetre), slightly larger partings can be used, but avoid stretching or pulling the hair towards the rod because this can cause hair breakage or straight, misdirected hair at the scalp.

Hair length and perming

Hair that is 5 cm to 15 cm (2 to 6 inches) long is considered ideal for perming. Hair should be long enough to make at least 2.5 turns around the rod. To perm hair longer than 15 cm (6 inches), smaller partings must be used to allow the waving lotion and neutraliser to penetrate more easily and thoroughly.

Perm lotion selection

The type of perm lotion you choose depends on the total evaluation of your client's hair and wishes during the consultation and pre-perm analysis. The following is a general guide to help you decide whether to use an alkaline or an acid-balanced perm.

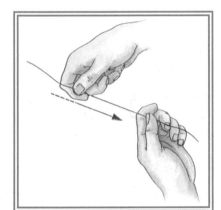

Figure 16.15 (a) Coarse; (b) Medium; (c) Fine

Figure 16.16 Testing for elasticity

Hair Type	Type of Perm Lotion
Coarse, resistant	Alkaline lotion wind or alkaline water wind
Fine, resistant	Alkaline lotion wind or alkaline water wind
Normal	Alkaline water wind or acid balanced
Normal, porous	Alkaline water wind or acid-balanced
Normal, delicate	Acid-balanced
Tinted, non-porous	Alkaline water wind or acid-balanced
Tinted, porous	Acid-balanced
Highlighted/frosted/ dimensionally coloured	Acid-balanced
Highlighted, tinted	Acid-balanced
Bleached	Acid-balanced

Today's perm products offer a wide selection of special features and formulas for all hair types. There are alkaline formulas for bleached hair and acid-balanced formulas for resistant hair. Each formula gives excellent results if you choose the perm carefully and follow the manufacturer's directions.

Pre-perm cutting or shaping

If your client has chosen a hairstyle that is the same or very similar to the design he or she is currently wearing, reshape the style using either a scissors or razor. If the finished style requires texturising or thinning of the ends, wait until after giving the perm to texturise. Over-tapered or thinned ends are more difficult to wrap smoothly and accurately. Irregular effects cut into hair can be difficult to wind without distortion of the hair. Lightly tapering thick hair before winding can aid the winding process. If your client wants a completely new style, rough cut the hair into an approximation of the final shape. After the perm is completed, you can finish shaping the style more exactly.

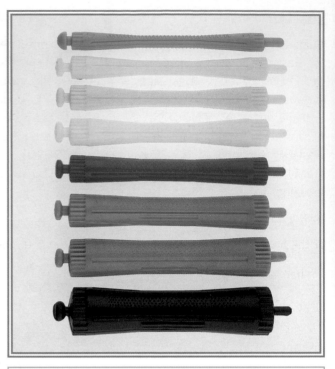

Figure 16.17 Perm curlers, or rods, colour coded according to size

Perm curlers and rods

Correct selection of perm curler size is essential for successful perm results. The size of curler controls/determines the size of curl created by the waving process. Perm curlers are typically made of plastic and come in varying sizes. They range in diameter (distance through the centre of the curler) from small to large (0.3 to 1.9 cm (⅛ to ¾")). Rods are usually colour coded to easily identify their size.

Perm curlers are also available in various lengths: short, medium and long (4.4 to 8.8 cm (1¾ to 3½")). Rods of all diameters are available in long lengths. Medium and short lengths are not always available in all diameters. These shorter curlers are used for wrapping small or awkward sections.

Remember: When selecting perm rods for use with acid perms, choosing one size smaller than the required curl size can help to reduce the effect of curl drop, sometimes experienced with this type of perm.

As well as the traditional shape of perm curler, there are a range of alternatives, some especially designed to achieve specific shapes in the hair. These include spiral curlers, rick-rack sticks, triangular curlers, flexible curlers and crimping shapers.

Types of curlers

There are two types of curlers: concave and straight. Concave curlers have a small diameter in the centre area and gradually increase to their largest diameter at the ends, resulting in a tighter curl at the hair ends, with a looser, wider curl at the scalp. The diameter of straight curlers is the same throughout their length, creating an even-sized curl from end to scalp.

All curlers have some means of securing the hair on the curler to prevent the curl from unwinding. Usually an elastic band, with a fastening button or loop attached to the end, stretches across the wound hair and secures it when the button or loop is inserted into the opposite end of the curler. Rounded curler rubbers are less likely to mark and break hair than flat ones.

Selecting rod size

When selecting curler size, two things must be considered:

- amount of curl desired
- physical characteristics of the hair.

Curl desired

The amount of wave, curl, or body needed is determined between you and your client during the consultation. Your success in creating a style depends primarily on the curler sizes you choose, the number of curlers used, and where the curlers are placed on the head.

Hair characteristics

Of the hair characteristics described earlier, three are important to curler size selection:

- hair length
- hair elasticity
- hair texture.

Suggested hair sectioning and curler size

Although the hair length, elasticity and texture must be considered in the choice of curlers, the texture should be the determining factor.

Coarse texture, good elasticity

Requires smaller (narrower) sections and larger curlers to permit better placement of curlers for a definite wave pattern.

Medium texture, average elasticity

Medium or average textured hair requires sections that are the same size as the size of the curler.

Fine texture, poor elasticity

Requires smaller sections and curlers wound without any tension on the hair.

Hair in nape area

Use short sections and short curlers.

Long hair

To permanently wave hair longer than 15 cm (6 inches), use small sections. This permits the waving lotion and neutraliser to penetrate more easily and thoroughly. Spiral winding, piggy back or double winding techniques may be used to achieve an even curl pattern from ends to scalp.

Pre-perm shampooing

Today, there are products specifically formulated for pre-perm shampooing that thoroughly yet gently cleanse the hair. Use of these shampoos is recommended for optimal results.

When analysing a client's hair before perming, you might notice that the hair looks and feels coated. This coating might be due to the build-up of shampoo or conditioners, improper rinsing, resins from styling products or hair spray, or mineral deposits from hard water. The coating can prevent penetration of the waving lotion and interfere with perm

Note: While shampooing or doing any pre-perm preparation of a client's hair, you should avoid vigorous brushing, combing, pulling or rubbing that can cause the scalp to become sensitive to perm solutions.

results. It is very important for the hair to be free of all coatings before beginning any perm.

Begin the process by wetting the hair, applying the shampoo, and gently working into a lather. If the hair is extremely coated let the shampoo remain in the hair for several minutes before rinsing. Rinse thoroughly to remove all shampoo and dissolved build-up. Towel blot excess water from the hair.

Sectioning and parting

Pre-sectioning is dividing the hair into uniform working areas at the top, front, crown, sides, back and nape. Pre-sectioning makes the work easier as it ensures that the curlers will fit onto the client's head in the direction that you intend. It also secures the hair out of the way and not on your client's face while winding.

Parting, also known as blocking, is the overall plan for the curler placement. You block so that you know where to place the curlers in order to give the design the support, direction and curl pattern it needs. It is important that the blocking is done in uniform sections. You should use the following guidelines to help you:

- uniformly arrange sections
- equally subdivide sections (blockings)
- create clean and uniform partings (length and width)
- the average parting should match the diameter (size) of the curler being used
- the length of the blocking should be the same as or a little shorter, but never longer, than the length of the curler (see Figures 16.18 – 16.20).

The perm wind/wrap

Winding/wrapping patterns

Just as the curler size and sectioning size determine the size of the curl, the winding pattern determines the direction or flow of the curl.

Popular winding patterns are:

- orthodox wind
- brick wind
- directional wind
- carousel wind
- spiral wind
- stack wind.
- octopus wind
- wind and leave
- pincurl perm
- piggy back wind

All winding patterns may be adapted to suit particular head shapes and to allow the blocking to follow the direction of the required hairstyle or the natural fall of the hair.

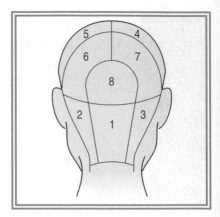

Figure 16.18 Sectioning

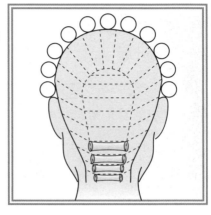

Figure 16.19 Blocking

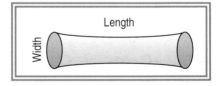

Figure 16.20 Length denotes span of blocking. Width refers to the depth of the blocking.

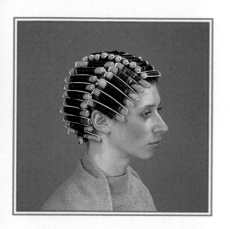

Figure 16.21 Orthodox wind

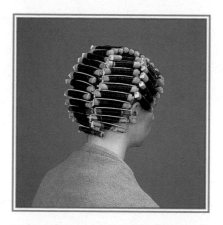

Figure 16.22 Orthodox wind

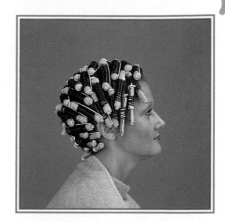

Figure 16.23 Brick wind

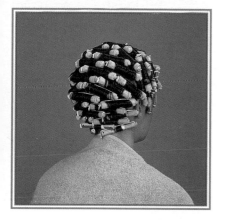

Figure 16.24 Brick wind

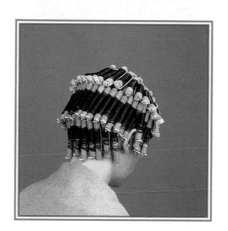

Figure 16.25 Directional wind

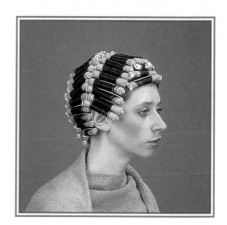

Figure 16.26 Directional wind

Orthodox (conventional) wind

This traditional sectioning pattern is perhaps the most widely used when perming. The hair is divided into nine sections to allow the curlers to fit easily on the head. This allows the curlers to be wound in a downward direction, following the natural fall of the hair and back off the face. The top/front section may also be wound in a forward direction if required to follow the direction of the hairstyle or to follow natural fall of the hair on the top.

Brick wind

This technique does not use pre-sectioning. The curlers are located on the head in a staggered brickwork pattern. This technique prevents the occurrence of continuous partings in the end curl pattern and makes the technique very suitable for use when perming hair that will be natural dried, especially short hair.

The wind commences at the focal point of the hairstyle, usually at the front. The skill of the hairdresser is to position the curlers in a brickwork pattern that will follow the direction of the required hairstyle

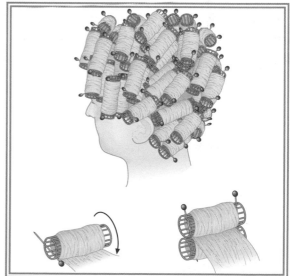

Figure 16.27 Spiral wind

Directional wind

Sectioning patterns may be devised to enable the curlers to fit onto the head in directions that will support the direction of the hairstyle. Pre-sectioning will ensure that all curlers fit onto the head without placing the hair under tension.

Carousel wind

This pattern will enable long hair to be wound on the ends, without perming the root area. This produces a wavy look on the hair without giving a too full a look to the head.

Spiral wind

This technique is used when a continuous curl is required along the length of long hair, without root lift. Pre-sectioning is essential when spiral winding as the wrap will hang down and obscure the scalp area below and therefore the wind works from the lower areas of the head first. Without sectioning the hair will be difficult to control.

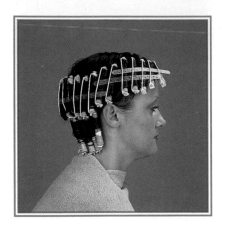

Figure 16.28 Carousel wind

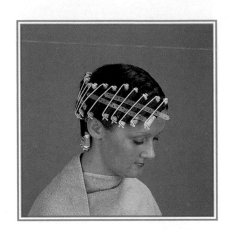

Figure 16.29 Carousel wind

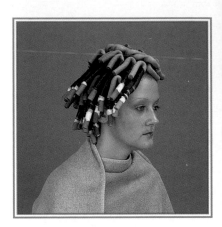

Figure 16.30 Spiral wind

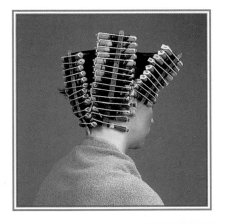

Figure 16.31 Stack wind

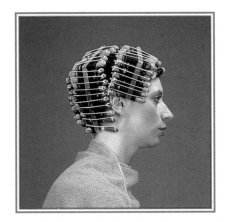

Figure 16.32 Inverted stack wind with stacking sticks

Stack wind

This technique may be used to produce curl at the ends of the hair. It may be used to produce a large volume at the ends of the hair, with a definite flatter area at the top of the head.

If the technique incorporates an inverted stack on the top of the head, an overall curl effect may be produced without producing a large level of volume on the top. It is very suitable for thick plentiful hair.

Octopus wind

This technique should be wound with lotion. It gives a natural-looking wave and curl with irregular volume and movement. Follow the direction of the style. Ensure that the rollers are placed on the base.

Take the section directly behind the first. Wind down the roller, slightly over directing in order to place the roller directly on top of the one sitting on its base. Use a plastic pin between the two rollers to secure both ends of the curlers. If you require irregular wave movement alternate the diameter size of the curlers.

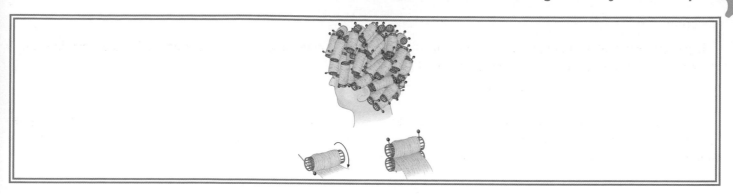

Figure 16.33 Octopus wind

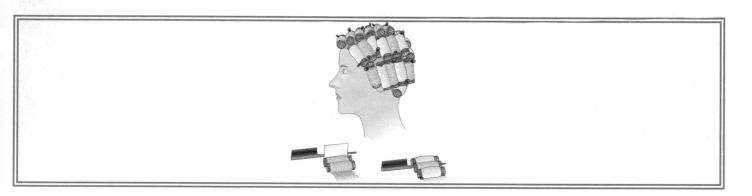

Figure 16.34 Wind and leave

Wind and leave

This technique gives volume with a soft curl. It is ideal for thick, coarse hair with a natural wave curl. You will need easi-meche or foil for this technique. Wind the hair without lotion alternating using easi-meshe or foil. Post-damp curlers that aren't covered. Neutralise as normal.

Pin curl perm

This technique can be used on short hair that requires a soft movement. It is also good on hair that is finer and longer, giving wave and movement but leaving it flatter on the top. You will need plastic pin curl clips. The hair is wound with lotion and directed into the style. Take triangular sections using end papers. You can make the pin curl movement vary by using the following formats:

- open middle – soft movement
- tighter middle – stronger curl movement
- barrel curl – lift at the root
- flat curl – flat at the root.

Alternate the pin curl direction of each row. A good shaped pin curl is vital for the success of this perm. Place a net over the pin curls when neutralising and do not have the water too powerful when rinsing so the curls are not disturbed.

The piggyback (double curler) wind

The piggyback (double curler) method of wrapping is especially suitable for extra long hair. This wrapping technique permits maximum control of the size and tightness of the curl from the scalp to the hair ends. Control of the amount of curl can be exercised by the size of the curlers selected. Thus, the use of larger curlers will result in a loose, wide wave;

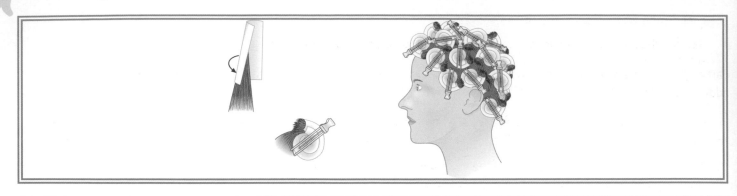

Figure 16.35 Pin curl perm

while small, or medium curlers will give tighter curls. The following is the procedure for wrapping in the piggyback (double curler) method:

1. Section the head in the usual manner (orthodox sectioning).

2. Select the desired size curlers. The curlers used in the midpoint to the scalp area should be at least one size larger than those used on the hair ends.

3. About halfway up the strand, place porous end papers one on top and one underneath.

4. Start at the midpoint part of the strand. Place the larger curler underneath the hair strand and start winding.

5. Roll the curler towards the scalp and, at the same time, control the hair ends by holding them to the left away from the rod.

6. Secure the wrapped curler at the scalp, leaving the hair ends dangling free from the rod.

7. Place an end paper on the hair strand covering the ends. Using the smaller size curler, wind the hair ends up to the above larger rod.

8. Secure the second rod to rest against the first one in piggyback fashion.

9. To maintain better control over the winding and processing, it is advisable to complete the winding of each strand before proceeding to the next one.

10. Test curls should be taken from the curlers closer to the scalp because the hair in this area is more resistant and might require additional processing.

When winding hair, always avoid bulkiness on the rod. Bulkiness prevents the formation of a good curl because the hair cannot conform to the shape of the curler, and the waving lotion and neutraliser cannot penetrate evenly and thoroughly. To ensure a smooth wave formation and avoid fishhook (buckled) ends, the first turn of the curler should be the end papers without any of the hair ends between them.

Piggyback wind (alternative method)

This technique avoids the distortion of the hair that can at times occur on the area between the two curlers. It does, however, create an elongated curl on the area of the hair nearest the scalp.

1. Locate the end papers at the ends of the hair and wind the ends of the hair with the smaller perm curler.

2. Wind the curler to a mid point of the hair length and then insert a second perm curler. Wind both curlers together to the scalp and secure.

Partial perming

Perming only a section of a whole head of hair is called partial perming. Partial perming can be used on:

- clients (male and female) who have long hair on the top and crown and very short, tapered sides and nape

- clients who need volume and lift only in certain areas
- designs that require curl support in the nape area but a smooth, sleek surface.

Partial perming uses the same techniques and wrapping patterns that have already been described. There are a few additional considerations:

- When you are winding the hair and reach the area that will be left unpermed, go to the next larger rod size so that the curl pattern of the permed hair will blend into the unpermed hair.
- After wrapping the area to be permed, place a coil of moist cotton wool around the wrapped rods as well as around the entire hairline
- Before applying the waving lotion, apply a heavy, creamy conditioner to the sections that will not be permed to protect this hair from the effects of the waving lotions (waving lotion softens and straightens unwrapped hair).

Winding/wrapping the hair

To create a uniform wave or curl pattern, the hair must be wrapped smoothly and cleanly on each perm curler without stretching. As noted earlier, the action of the waving lotion expands the hair. Hair that is tightly wrapped interferes with this action, damaging the hair, and preventing penetration of the waving lotion and neutraliser.

When winding with acid wave a slight tension may be used.

Hair strand parting in relation to the head

The term 'base' refers to the area of the head or scalp where the curler is placed in relation to the head. The curlers can be wrapped on-base, off-base, or one-half off-base. Each of these curler positions creates a slightly different scalp wave direction, which will influence the overall curl pattern results.

Curl on-base

When the strand is held in an upward position (90 degrees to the head) and wound on the rod, the curl will rest on-base (see Figure 16.36). Hair wound in this manner will produce curls that start close to the scalp for hairstyles that require fullness, height and upward movement. When perming very curly hair, over directing the hair (holding the hair at more than 90 degrees to the head) will enable control of the curl even closer to the scalp.

Curl off-base

When the strand is held in a downward position and wound on a curler, the curl will rest off-base (see Figure 16.37). Hair wound in this manner will produce a curl that starts further away from the scalp (root drag), than hair wound on-base. Off-base winding produces close-to-the-head hairstyles that do not require fullness of height.

Curl one-half off-base

When the strand is held straight out from the head and wound on a curler, the curl will rest one-half off-base (see Figure 16.38). Hair wound in this manner is adaptable to many styles.

End papers

End papers or end tissues are porous papers used to cover the ends of the hair to ensure smooth and even wrapping. End papers minimise the danger of buckled or

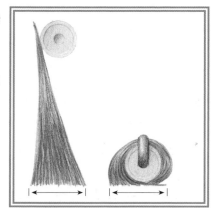

Figure 16.36 Curl on-base

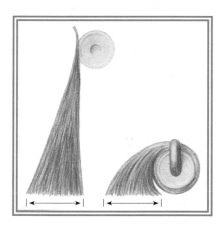

Figure 16.37 Curl off-base

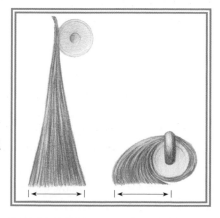

Figure 16.38 Curl one-half off-base

distorted ends and help to form smooth, even curls and waves. They are especially important in helping to wrap uneven hair lengths smoothly.

There are three methods of end paper application in general use today. Each method is equally effective, if properly used:

- double end paper wrap
- single end paper wrap
- book end wrap.

Hair should be shampooed and left moist (not saturated) for wrapping. Section hair and begin by making your first parting. Remember, each parting should be no longer than the length of the curler. If the parting is too long, the hair will not wave evenly and hair may be placed under undue tension. If the hair should become dry while you are winding, moisten the hair lightly using water from a trigger spray.

Directions:

1 *Part off and comb the parted hair up and out until all the hair is smooth and evenly distributed. Do not pinch the ends together.*

2 *Place one end paper under the hair strand so that it extends below the ends of the hair. Place the other end paper on the top.*

3 *With your right hand, place the curler under the double end papers, parallel with the parting at the scalp.*

4 *Wind the strand smoothly on the curler to the scalp without tension.*

5 *Fasten the band on the top of the curler.*

Note: To prevent breakage, the band should not press into the hair near the scalp or be twisted (flat rubbers) against the wound hair.

Double end paper wrap

The preparation and winding of curls for a single end paper wrap and book end wrap are the same as the double end paper wrap, with the following exceptions:

Single end paper wrap

Place only one end paper on top of the hair strand and hold it flat between the first and second fingers to prevent bunching. The hair is wound in the same manner as the double end paper wrap.

Book end wrap

Hold the strand between the first and second fingers; fold and place end paper over the strand, forming an envelope. Take care not to indent into the hair with the folded side of the paper. Wind the curl as in the double end paper wrap.

Applying waving lotion

Styles of application

Pre-saturation

May be used when perming strong straight hair. By applying the lotion to all of the hair before commencing winding, the hair begins to soften, uniformly, and offers less resistance to winding.

Pre-damping

Wetting the hair with perm lotion as you wind. This enables more resistant areas, if wound first, to begin to soften before the less resistant, therefore producing an even curl development throughout the head. This method may also be used when perming hair using winding patterns to which it may be difficult to apply the perm lotion after winding. In some cases a mild lotion strength may be used as a wrapping lotion, followed by a stronger lotion, post-damping. This is often used when perming hair with differing rates of porosity along the hair's length.

Post-damping

The hair is water wound, and then the lotion is applied after the wind is completed. This gives time for the winding process to take place. Care must be taken to ensure lotion is applied to all wound curlers.

> **Remember:** *Whenever winding with perm lotion, either pre-saturation or pre-damping, wear protective gloves to protect your skin.*

After shampooing, shaping and wrapping the hair, place a coil or band of cotton wool moistened with water around the entire hairline. To prevent skin irritation and for added protection, apply a barrier cream to skin around the hairline before applying the cotton band. This safety precaution prevents waving lotion from coming into contact with the skin and possibly causing irritation. If lotion is applied accurately there should be a minimum of dripping, but the cotton is assurance of your client's comfort and safety. After the waving lotion has been applied remove the cotton wool, gently pat the skin with water-soaked cotton wool, and replace with fresh.

Unless otherwise specified in the product instruction, apply waving lotion with care to the wound hair. Systematically apply lotion to each curler, in turn, using an applicator bottle. Run the nozzle along the top of the curler, releasing lotion onto the hair. Avoid allowing lotion to flood onto the scalp. Coverage will be assured by making three applications to the entire head, a little at a time. Remember, dry hair will not absorb moisture easily. By gradually adding lotion to the hair it will more readily absorb ensuring thorough distribution and coverage.

> **Remember:** *Should perm lotion enter your client's eyes, rinse with sterile water from an eye bath. Should eye irritation continue, inform your line manager and if required seek medical advice.*

Processing time

Processing time is the length of time required for the hair strands to absorb the waving lotion (softening) and for the hair to re-curl (rearrangement of chemical bonds). It depends on the hair type (porosity, elasticity, length, density, texture and overall condition) and the specific perm you are using. Again, follow the manufacturer's directions explicitly. It is usually safe to anticipate the processing time to be less than suggested by the manufacturer or a client's previous record card. Some perms have stop-action processing so that all you have to do is set a timer. Some perms give you a general timetable to follow and require that you do a test curl during processing. It is very important to time the perm process accurately to help prevent over or under processing.

The ability of the hair to absorb moisture may vary from time to time in the same individual, even when the same lotions and procedures are used. A record of the previous processing time is desirable, but should be used only as a guide.

It is sometimes necessary to saturate all the curlers a second time during the processing time. This might be due to:

- evaporation of the lotion or dryness of the hair
- hair poorly saturated by the hair stylist
- no wave development after the maximum time indicated by the manufacturer
- improper selection of solution strength for the client's hair
- failure to follow the manufacturer's directions for a specific formula.

A reapplication of the lotion will hasten processing. Watch the wave development closely. Negligence can result in hair damage.

Most manufacturers provide instructions with their product. Here are some you will encounter:

- 'Process at room temperature'. Make sure that your client is not sitting in a draught or too close to a heater. A room that is cool slows down the processing time.
- 'Place a plastic cap over the wrapped curlers'. Be sure that the plastic cap covers all the curlers and that the cap is airtight. Secure the cap with a non-metallic clip. The cap holds in scalp heat. If it is too loose or if all the rods are not

covered, processing might take longer. A dry towel placed over the plastic cap will increase the effect and will reduce the influence of blasts of warm or cold air on parts of the head (producing uneven development).

- 'Preheated dryer'. Turn the hood dryer to a high setting and medium air flow. Allow the dryer to warm up for approximately five minutes before placing your client under the dryer. Cover the wound curlers with a plastic cap secured in place, locate the hood to enclose all of the curlers and reduce the heat to a medium setting. (Note: Dryer filters should be cleaned frequently so that optimum heat and airflow will remain constant). Take care not to overprocess the hair, in particular porous hair.

- 'Accelerator, climazone or rollerball'. This may be used to aid the process of the perm. The curlers are not usually covered with a plastic cap, the heater must be located correctly and evenly around the head. Using the correct heat setting process, taking care not to allow the hair to become dry. In some cases these machines are programmable to particular lotions and hair types. Having located a sensor on the hair it will regulate the processing.

Testing curls during processing

Optimum curl development occurs only once during the processing time. The ability to read a test curl 'S' formation and recognise proper wave development will help you avoid two of the most common problems in perming: over processing and under processing. Three test curls should be taken: in the nape, on top of the head and on the side of the head. These three locations will allow you to judge the progress of curl development on the most resistant and the least resistant areas of the head.

Water rinsing

Rinsing the waving lotion from the hair is extremely important. Any lotion left in the hair can cause poor perm results. When your test curl indicates that the optimum curl has been achieved, remove the cotton wool from around the hairline. Rinse the hair thoroughly with a moderate force of warm water. The manufacturer's perm directions will indicate how long you should rinse – usually three to five minutes. Always set your timer for the exact time. Remember, you are rinsing the lotion out of the internal hair structure, not merely off the surface. Make sure that all curlers are thoroughly rinsed. Pay special attention to the curlers at the nape of the neck. They are a little difficult to reach, but they must be rinsed as well as all the other curlers. Long hair and thick hair usually require the maximum rinsing time (five minutes) to make sure that all lotion has been removed from all hair wrapped around the curlers. Indicator papers are available which, when pressed to the hair, will indicate if any perm lotion remains in the hair.

Undesirable effects of improper or incomplete rinsing include:

- Early curl relaxation. Even if the perm has been processed correctly, any waving lotion left in the hair can interfere with the action of the neutraliser. If the neutraliser is not able to properly re-bond the hair, the curl will be weak or will not last very long.

- Lightening of hair colour (natural or tint). Rinsing helps reduce the pH of the hair and helps to close the cuticle layer. If the hair is not rinsed properly, the hydrogen peroxide in the neutraliser can react with waving lotion left in the hair and cause the hair colour to lighten. This lightening effect is usually seen on the hair ends.

- Residual perm odour. If any waving lotion is left in the hair, it will become trapped inside the hair when the neutraliser is applied. This is especially true of acid-balanced perms. Unpleasant odours may be evident each time the hair gets wet or damp.

Blotting after water rinsing

Careful blotting ensures that the neutraliser will penetrate the hair immediately and completely: do not omit this important step. To obtain the best results from towel blotting, carefully press a towel between each curler, using your fingers. Do not rock or roll the rods while blotting. When the hair is in a softened state, any such movement can cause hair breakage. Change to dry towels frequently in order to remove as much excess water as possible. Excess water left in the hair can dilute or weaken the action of the neutraliser. If this happens the curl can be either weak or relaxed. After rinsing and blotting has been completed, place a fresh clean band of cotton around the hairline before applying neutraliser.

Neutralising/normalising

Neutralising procedures can vary according to the perm product you are using. Again, follow the manufacturer's directions explicitly.

> **Remember:** Whenever handling perming chemicals, wear protective overalls and protective rubber gloves.

In general, the following procedure is the accepted method of neutralising:

1 Apply neutraliser to the top and underside of the rods. Apply to the top of the rod, then gently turn the rod up and apply to the underside of the rod in the same manner you applied the waving lotion. When using foam neutraliser, apply the neutraliser to the curlers and foam up.

2 Repeat the entire application a second time, to ensure complete coverage.

3 Wait five minutes to allow for optimum re-bonding. Set a timer for accuracy.

4 Remove the curlers carefully and gently, unwinding without tension as it may straighten the hair.

5 Work the remaining neutraliser onto the ends of the hair, pushing the neutraliser onto the hair so as not to drag the curl.

6 Rinse the hair thoroughly with warm water and apply an after-perm treatment if required.

7 Towel blot the hair and, using a wide tooth comb, gently comb the hair into place.

If you are uncertain of the procedure or whether an after-perm treatment should be applied, consult with your supervisor or stylist.

Post-perm precautions

After blotting, your new perm is ready for final shaping and styling. It is important to avoid shampooing, conditioning, stretching or excessive manipulations of freshly permed hair. When styling, do not pull on the hair or use intense heat that could result in curl relaxation. Generally, hair should not be shampooed, conditioned, or treated harshly for 48 hours after perming. This special care will help to ensure that the perm does not relax.

Ten pointers for a perfect perm

- Consult with your client.
- Analyse the hair and scalp carefully.
- Select the correct curler size for the desired style.
- Choose the appropriate perm product for the hair type and final design. Follow the manufacturer's directions carefully.
- Section and make accurate partings for each curler. Wrap specifically for the style chosen.
- Apply waving lotion to the top and underside of all wound curlers, one at a time. Ensure each curler is thoroughly wet with lotion.
- If the perm product requires a test curl, be sure the result is a firmly formed 'S' shape.
- Water rinse for at least three to five minutes and carefully towel blot each curler.
- Apply neutraliser to the top and underside of all curlers. Saturate thoroughly. Wait

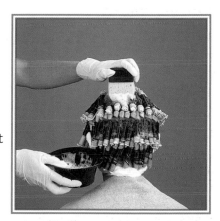

Figure 16.39 Applying foam neutraliser

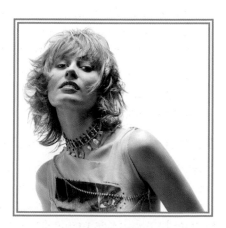

Figure 16.40

five minutes, remove the curler carefully, without pulling, apply remaining neutraliser, and gently work through the hair. Rinse with warm water.

● Educate your client in how to care for their new look. Recommend hair care and styling products that are suitable. Instruct in how best to style the hair at home and remind your client not to shampoo the hair for at least 24 hours and to avoid getting the hair wet during that period.

Clean up

● Discard all used materials.

● Clean up the work area.

● Thoroughly clean and sterilise the curlers and other tools used.

● Wash and dry your hands.

● Complete your client's record card.

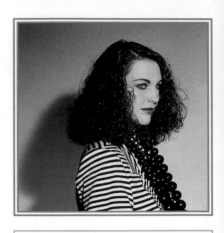

Figure 16.41

Alternative (unconventional) perming techniques

The curl shape and structure achieved using conventional perm rods with traditional (croquignole) winding techniques will usually be uniform in its appearance. The only exception is directional winding, which is possible with conventional rods. For special perming techniques you need to use alternative perming systems. Here are some examples.

Spiral rods

Directions:

1 *Take a small rectangular section of hair.*
2 *Place a rod hook over the hair and slide it towards the scalp.*
3 *Wind the hair around the rod.*
4 *Secure the ends with a spiral clip.*
5 *Repeat steps 1–4 to complete the entire head.*

Foam rollers and formers

Directions:

1 *Take a small rectangular section of hair.*
2 *Secure the hair points in an end paper.*
3 *Wind the hair around the roller.*
4 *Secure the roller by bending it over.*
5 *Repeat steps 1–4 to complete the entire head.*

Crimpers

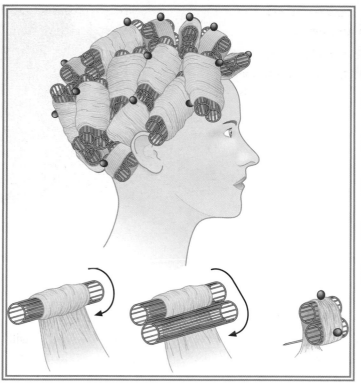

Figure 16.42 The double-decker wind

Directions:

1 Take a conventional winding hair section, no wider than the rimpers.

2 Place the open crimper, with its spikes facing upwards, under the hair section.

3 Place an end paper on the ends of the hair section and close the crimper.

4 Depending on the hair length, continue with extra crimpers.

5 Repeat steps 1–4 to complete the entire head.

Chopsticks

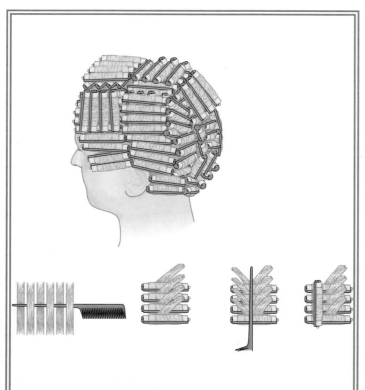

Figure 16.43 The hopscotch wind

Directions:

1 Take a small square section of hair and protect it with one or more end papers.

2 Place the hair section through the loop and hold it securely.

3 Separate the chopstick 'legs' and wind the hair in a figure of eight.

4 Secure the end paper on to the chopsticks using a rubber band.

5 Repeat steps 1–4 to complete the entire head.

U-stick rods

Directions:

1 *Take a small square section of hair and pull it through the middle of the U-stick.*

2 *Wind the hair in a figure-of-eight movement around the U-stick.*

3 *Protect the ends with one or more end papers.*

4 *Secure the end papers on the U-stick with a rubber band.*

5 *Repeat steps 1–4 to complete the entire head.*

Preliminary (pre-perm) test curls

Preliminary test curls help determine how your client's hair will react to a perm. It is advisable to carry out a test on hair that is tinted, bleached, over-porous, or shows any signs of damage.

Remember: When applying perm lotion you should wear protective gloves or apply barrier cream to your hands.

Preliminary testing gives you the following additional information:

● Actual processing time needed to achieve optimum curl results.

● Curl results based on the curler size and perm product you have selected.

Directions:

1 *Shampoo the hair and towel dry.*

2 *Following the perm direction, wrap two or three curlers in the most delicate areas of the hair.*

3 *Wind a coil of cotton around the curler.*

4 *Apply waving lotion to the wrapped curls, being careful not to allow the waving lotion to come in contact with the unwrapped hair.*

5 *Set a timer and process the hair according to the perm directions.*

6 *Check the hair frequently.*

To check a test curl, unfasten a rod and carefully (remember – hair is in a softened state) unwind the curl about one-and-a-half turns of the curler. Do not permit the hair to become loose or unwound from the curler completely. Hold the hair firmly by placing a thumb at each end of the curler. Move the curler gently towards the scalp so that the hair falls loosely into the wave pattern. Continue checking the curlers until a firm and definite 'S' is formed. The 'S' reflects the size of the rod used. Be guided by the manufacturer's directions.

When judging test curls, different hair textures with varying degrees of elasticity will have slightly different 'S' formations. Fine, thin hair is generally softer and has less bulk. The wave ridge might be less defined and more difficult to read. Coarse, thick hair has better elasticity and seems to reinforce itself, falling into wave pattern more readily. The wave ridge will be stronger and better defined. Long hair may produce a wider scalp wave than short hair, because larger curlers are used and the diameter of the wave widens towards the scalp.

When the optimum curl has been formed, rinse the curls with warm water, blot the curls thoroughly, apply, process and rinse the neutraliser according to the perm directions and gently dry these test curls. Evaluate the curl results. If the hair is over-processed, do not perm the rest of the hair until it is in better condition. If the test curl results are good, proceed with the perm, but do not re-perm these preliminary test curls.

Overprocessing

Any lotion that can properly process the hair can also overprocess it, causing dryness, frizziness or hair damage. Overprocessed hair is easily detected. It cannot be combed into a suitable wave pattern, because the elasticity of the hair has been excessively damaged, and the hair feels harsh after being dried. Reconditioning treatments should begin immediately.

Causes of over processing are:

- Lotion left on the hair too long.
- Improperly judged pre-perm hair analysis and/or waving lotion that was too strong.
- Test curls were not made frequently enough or were judged improperly.

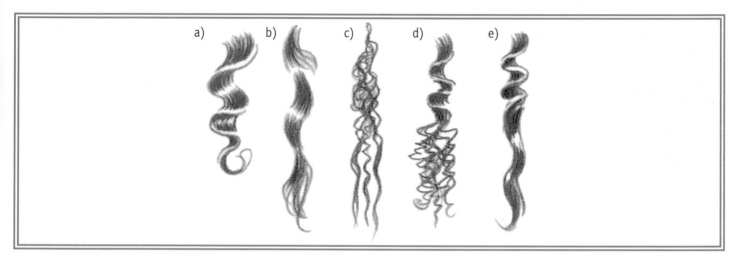

Figure 16.44 (a) Good results; (b) Underprocessed curl; (c) Overprocessed curl; (d) Porous ends; (e) Improper winding

Underprocessing

Underprocessing is caused by insufficient processing time of the waving lotion. After perming, underprocessed hair has a limp or weak wave formation. The ridges are not well defined, and the hair retains little or no wave formation. Typically, after a few shampooings, the hair will have no curl pattern at all (see Figure 16.44).

Underprocessed hair, even if there is no curl, has been chemically treated. If, in your professional judgement, you decide the hair can be re-permed, condition it first, choose a milder lotion, and test the curl development frequently.

Problems and solutions

Problem	Possible Cause	Immediate Action	Future Action
Hair damage, breakage	Too much tension on hair, curlers too tight. Hair overprocessed; chemicals too strong	Apply restructurant or deep-action conditioner to remainder of the hair	Use less tension. Review choice of lotion, timing, etc. Do not re-perm
Scalp burn	Perm lotion flooding the scalp. Tension on the hair too excessive	Treat as a chemical burn. Rinse thoroughly with cool/tepid water. Refer to doctor if needed	Make a record to ensure the following points are used when the client's scalp is clear – use less tension; apply lotion to hair and not to the scalp
Sore hairline, skin irritation	Chemicals have been allowed to come into contact with the skin. Poor scalp ventilation	Consult the client regarding allergies. Rinse the scalp thoroughly. Apply soothing lotion but make sure the client is not allergic to it. Refer to doctor if the condition is serious	Consult the client regarding allergies, etc. Keep the lotion off the skin. Do not leave cotton wool around the hairline once the lotion has been applied. Use cotton wool with water to help dilute any lotion
Straight frizz	Lotion is too strong for the hair. Excessive winding tension. Hair overprocessed	Cut off ends to reduce frizz. Apply restructurant or penetrating conditioner	Ensure appropriate lotion is used in the future. Wind with less tension. Time carefully. Do not perm until all the old perm is cut out
Perm result too curly	Misunderstood client's request. Curlers too small. Lotion too strong	Depending on the condition relax the hair to reduce the curl using Silk straight European Curl for sensitised hair	Ensure appropriate lotion and curlers are used. Consultation prior to the process
No result	Lotion too weak or not used enough. Curlers too large. Poor neutralising. Hair underprocessed. Hair too wet when applying lotion Wrong pre-perm shampoo/conditioner used	If the hair condition allows, re-perm with suitable lotion, usually weaker than the first time	Use appropriate lotion and rods. Make sure you use a pre-perm shampoo
Fish-hooks	Hair points not wrapped properly. No end papers	Remove ends by cutting	Check points of hair are wrapped correctly. Use end papers
Perm weakness – amount of curl lessens over time	Poor neutralising. Hair stretched excessively while drying	If hair condition allows, re-perm with suitable lotion, usually weaker than the first time	Check method and timing of neutralising and perm lotion
Uneven curl	Uneven perm winding technique. Uneven tension. Uneven lotion application. Ineffective neutralising	If hair condition allows, re-perm with suitable lotion, usually weaker than the first time	Check tension of curlers before applying perm lotion or neutraliser
Good result when wet, poor when dry	Overprocessed	Apply conditioning agents to restructure the hair	Check method and timing of neutraliser and perm lotion
Straight pieces	Lotion not applied evenly. Rods too large	If the hair condition allows, re-perm affected area (always use a weaker strength of lotion than the first time	Ensure even lotion application

There are various perm lotions available especially designed for today's creative perming techniques. Indola, Wella, L'Oreal, Goldwell etc. have a range of products for all types of curl result and hair types. These are just a few examples:

- Indola do a modern ACID BALANCED permanent waving lotion with Silkquat Complex.

  A – Sensitive, normal and resistant hair.

  B – Coloured, highlighted and bleached hair.

- Silkwave Respective is a modern ALKALINE permanent styling lotion

  A – Resistant hair.

  B – Normal hair.

  C – Coloured hair.

- Valore is a high quality, self-balancing advanced perm formulation for perfect results and longer lasting curl retention.

  Ampholitic Foaming Agent allows penetration with non-aggressive action.

  Cationic Polymers give lightly conditioned curls that reinforce the hair and aid de-tangling

  A – Natural difficult hair.

  B – Natural hair.

  C – Tinted or porous hair.

Important safety precautions

Remember that the lotions used for perming contain chemically active ingredients and must therefore be used carefully to avoid injury to you and your client. The following precautions should always be taken:

- Protect your client's clothing with a plastic shampoo cape.
- Ask your client to remove glasses, earrings and necklaces to prevent damage.
- Do not undertake a perm on a client who has experienced an allergic reaction to a previous perm.
- Do not save any opened, unused waving lotion or neutraliser. These lotions can change in strength and effectiveness if not used within a few hours of opening the container.
- Do not dilute or add anything to the waving lotion or neutraliser unless the product directions tell you to do so.
- Keep waving lotion out of the eyes and away from the skin. If waving lotion should contact these areas, rinse thoroughly with cool clean water.
- Do not perm and apply hair colour to a client on the same day. Perm the hair first, wait one week, then apply hair colour. However, there are products available that combine perming and colouring within the one process.

Additional information

Useful websites

Website Addresses	Content
www.habia.org.uk	Hairdressing and Beauty Industry Authority. Downloads available including references to other websites
www.bbc-safety.co.uk	Free advice on health and safety
www.haircouncil.org.uk	UK statutory body for hairdressing
www.lookfantastic.com	Professional hairdressing products and advice
www.laurandp.co.uk	Educational publications for development of professional hairdressing
www.scott999.fsnet.co.uk	Hairdressing product information
www.nexus.com	Range of hairdressing products
www.tigi.co.uk	Range of hairdressing products
www.schwarzkopf.com	Range of hairdressing products
www.trichologists.org.uk	Institute of Trichologists

Magazines and journals

- *Hairdressers Journal*
- *Creative Head*
- *Estetica/Cutting Edge*
- *Black Beauty and Hair*

The evidence from the activities below will cover the Underpinning Knowledge for the Technical Certificate for Advanced Modern Apprenticeships. You will need to take the external test and carry out the practical activities (see City and Guilds Diploma Hairdressing 6915).

ACTIVITY

Outcome 1

Produce evidence for your portfolio on the following:

- *Describe how perm tests are carried out and how the tests can influence the perm service.*
- *Describe the effect of perm lotion and neutraliser on the hair structure.*
- *Describe the effect of temperature on the perming process.*
- *State when and why pre- and post-perm treatments should be used.*
- *Describe the types and causes of problems that may occur during the perming and neutralising process and how to correct them. Problems: hair/scalp damage (breakage, pull burns, sore hairline and skin irritation), perm too curly, fish hooks, good result when wet but poor result when dry, uneven curl, hair discoloured, curl drops after one to two weeks.*

- *State different types of perm lotions available and when they should be used for best effect.*

- *State what factors need to be considered when perming hair. Factors: client requirements, hair texture, hair growth and curl patterns, haircut and length, temperature, hair density, hair condition, hair structure, direction degree and extent of movement required.*

- *Describe the effect of different sectioning and winding techniques, and when they can be used for best effect.*

- *State the importance and effect of pH balance on the hair.*

- *Outline the Control of Substances Hazardous to Health Regulations 1999 (including subsequent amendments) and explain how they relate to perming products.*

- *State the importance of using personal protective equipment when perming.*

- *Describe the range of current fashion perm looks for men and women.*

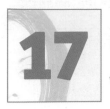

17 UNIT H30 COLOUR HAIR USING A VARIETY OF TECHNIQUES

1 Maintain effective and safe methods of working when colouring hair

2 Prepare for colouring

3 Create a variety of colouring effects

4 Resolve basic colouring problems

CHAPTER CONTENTS

- *Understanding Colour*
- *The International Colour Code*
- *Consultation and Diagnostics Prior to Colouring*
- *Contraindications When Using Permanent Tint*
- *Health and Safety When Colouring Hair*
- *Temporary Colours*

- *Semi-permanent Colours*
- *Permanent Oxidation Colour*
- *Quasi-permanent Colour*
- *Faults and Corrections*
- *Bleaching Principles*
- *Hydrogen Peroxide*
- *Colouring Techniques*

Understanding colour

Colouring is one of the most exciting areas in hairdressing and can be used in many ways but first you need to understand colour properly. Read through this information just to ensure you haven't forgotten anything.

Professional hair colours are made up of primary and secondary colours. All colours are derived from the three primary colours red, yellow and blue.

The secondary colours are achieved when a combination of primary colours are mixed together, for example:

- red + yellow = orange
- yellow + blue = green
- blue + red = violet

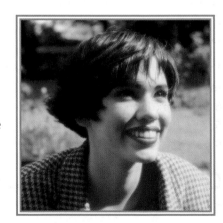

Figure 17.1

The colour circle shows the primary and secondary colours. Colours that are opposite will neutralise each other, e.g. to neutralise unwanted red tones you should apply a colour with an ash tone (blue).

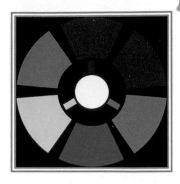

The International Colour Code

- Depth is the amount of pigment in the hair, e.g. how light or dark the hair is.
- Tone is the colour pigment that determines the character, e.g. Ash, Gold, Copper, etc.

The first number indicates depth, for example:

International colour chart	Depth	Colour	Tone
1/0	Blue black	/0	Natural
2/0	Black	/1	Special Ash
3/0	Dark Brown	/2	Cool Ash
4/0	Medium Brown	/3	Honey Gold
5/0	Light Brown	/4	Red
6/0	Dark Blonde	/5	Purple
7/0	Medium Blonde	/6	Violet
8/0	Light Blonde	/7	Brunette
9/0	Very Light Blonde	/8	Pearl Ash
10/0	Extra Light Blonde	/9	Soft Ash

Figure 17.2 The colour circle

The number after the point indicates the tone, e.g.

.0 Matt   .4 Copper
.1 Ash   .5 Mahogany
.2 Pearl   .6 Red
.3 Gold   .7 Violet

The first colour after the point is called the primary tone, the second is the secondary tone, e.g.

6   Dark Blonde
6.4.   Dark Copper Blonde
6.46   Dark Copper Red Blonde

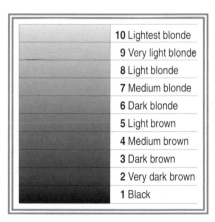

	10 Lightest blonde
	9 Very light blonde
	8 Light blonde
	7 Medium blonde
	6 Dark blonde
	5 Light brown
	4 Medium brown
	3 Dark brown
	2 Very dark brown
	1 Black

Figure 17.3 Natural hair colour levels

Consultation and diagnostics prior to colouring

Colours can be divided into two groups:

1. Cold shades (Ash, Matt – blues, greens, etc.)
2. Warm shades (Reds, Golds, etc.)

The cold shades will give an illusion of a darker colour, whilst warm shades appear lighter.

Always use a shade chart when selecting a colour with a client.

Remember:
- *Gold tones reflect light, making the final result appear lighter.*
- *Ash colours absorb the light, making the colours appear flatter and darker.*
- *When using an Ash tone remember that the result may appear deeper due to the ash tone.*

When the desired colour has been chosen it is your job as a hairdresser to consider the following:

- Ensure your client has had a skin test and check the results. This must be carried out 24–48 hours prior to colouring.

- Natural base colour. This will determine the strength of hydrogen peroxide to be used.

- Complexion and age of client. If incorrect or unsuitable colour has been chosen by the client advise accordingly but be tactful!

- Texture and density. If the hair is thick and abundant, tints will appear darker as less light shines through. Fine hair absorbs colour more quickly so less development time may be needed.

- Condition and porosity. A roughened hair shaft (open cuticle) will absorb colour more quickly. This means the hair is porous and soaks up colour rapidly so a shade or two lighter may be required.

  If the roots and middle lengths are in good condition stick to the original colour selection, but if the ends are porous emulsify the remaining tint once development time is complete. Work through to the ends, monitoring closely to avoid too much absorption. Virgin hair is hair that does not have traces of chemical processes on it.

- Tensile strength. Take a test cutting. If in doubt, do not proceed.

- Amount of white hair present. When a high percentage of white hair is present at the front of the head and is largely dark at the back it may be necessary to use different strengths of hydrogen peroxide, e.g. if a base 7 was desired (light blonde), 20 volume would be used to add colour to the front where the hair has a high percentage of white hair and 30 volume would be used at the back where the hair would be a natural base 5. This would give a 2/3 shades of lift. The term canities is used to describe white or colourless hair.

Contraindications when using permanent tint

If the client consultation results in any of the following contraindications, do not proceed with the service.

- The client has a contagious disease of the hair or scalp, e.g. ringworm, impetigo.

- Incompatible chemicals are present on the hair, i.e. metallic dyes.

- A positive reaction to a skin test.

- A lighter shade is required on previously tinted hair; this must be stripped out or lightened. Remember tint will not lift tint.

- Hair is weak and fragile (tensile strength).

Information about tests is included in Units G1 and G9, including skin tests, colour tests, porosity tests, elasticity tests, incompatibility tests and strand tests.

Health and safety when colouring hair

The Control of Substances Hazardous to Health (1992) Act (COSHH): includes the care, storing and handling of hazardous substances, for example:

- peroxides must be stored in a cool and dark area, either a metal cupboard away from heat and sunlight, or in a refrigerator

- bleaching and colouring products must be stored out of direct sunlight

- used products must be flushed away with water.

Care of self and others

- Personal protection; protective salon wear and plastic gloves.

- Client care; gown, plastic cape and towel or as per salon policy.

- Always read manufacturer's instructions or ask your trainer.

- Use tools and equipment carefully to avoid accidents.

- Ensure colour removal is done with care and with consideration to client comfort. Ensure the client is correctly positioned at the basin and that client protection is in place.

- Mop up any spillages.

- Report and record any accidents in The Accident Report Book.

- Ensure client record cards are completed correctly and stored in a safe place. Remember data protection, see Unit G9.

- Unsolved problems must be referred to your manager/trainer.

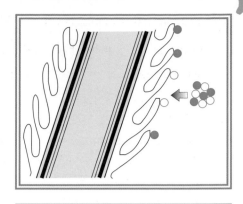

Figure 17.4 The action of temporary hair colour

Temporary colours

Temporary colours are a mild form of colour that last between one and five shampoos, depending on the porosity of the hair. A wide range of colours are available and they can be used as an introduction to colour. Temporary colours provide subtle toning to grey, white or naturally coloured hair and can be used to produce fashion effects on bleached hair.

Types of temporary colours

Temporary colours are available in the following mediums:

- Mousses
- Hairsprays
- Setting lotions
- Gels
- Glitter dust
- Creams

The chemistry of temporary colours

- Large colour molecules adhere to the outside of the cuticle and will not penetrate further into the hair as no hydrogen peroxide is used.

- Natural hair colour is not affected – there is no regrowth.

- However, unevenly porous hair can trap the colour molecules if the cuticle is open. Porosity equalisers can be used prior to applying temporary colours to smooth the cuticle surface.

Semi-permanent colours

Semi-permanent colours will last between six and eight shampoos. They only darken and tone and the colour gradually fades out.

Semi-permanent colours cover a small percentage of white hair. They come in a variable colour range and are generally ammonia free. Heat and porosity will accelerate development. A knowledge of consultation and colour selection is essential prior to use.

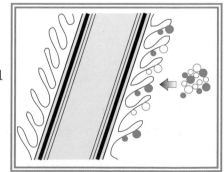

Figure 17.5 The action of semi-permanent hair colour formula

Advantages

- Excellent for conditioning hair.

- No mixing required.

- No regrowth visible.

- Skin tests are not usually required (read manufacturer's instructions).

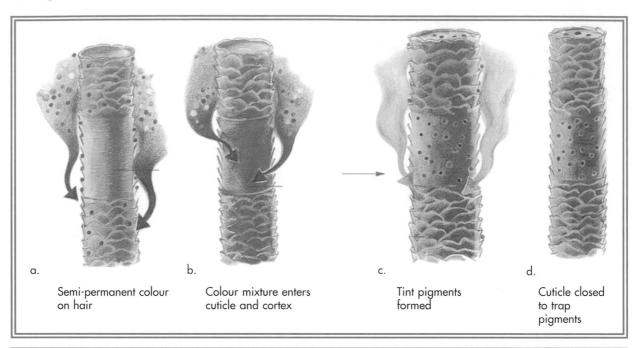

a.	b.	c.	d.
Semi-permanent colour on hair	Colour mixture enters cuticle and cortex	Tint pigments formed	Cuticle closed to trap pigments

Figure 17.6 Action of semi-permanent hair colours

- Quick and easy application.

- Clients can change hair colour frequently and easily without undue stress on the hair.

- Foaming action prevents dripping.

The chemistry of semi-permanent colours

- Small colour molecules penetrate the cuticle layers and enter the cortex.

- They are gradually removed each time the hair is shampooed as the water pushes some of the molecules out.

Permanent oxidation colour

These are the most popular type of colour in professional hairdressing. They are available in a wide variety of permanent colours that give full coverage of natural and white hair. They are developed in creams, gels and liquid form and are mixed with hydrogen peroxide or another oxidant. They will darken, lighten and tone. Highlight tints mixed with developer or 40 vol/12% hydrogen peroxide are used when four shades of lift are required.

Remember: A skin test is essential 24 hours prior to treatment.

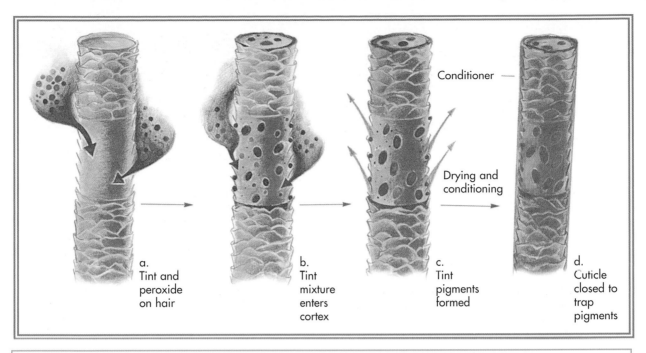

Figure 17.7 (a) Tint and peroxide on hair; (b) Tint mixture enters cortex; (c) Tint pigments formed; (d) Cutic

The chemistry of permanent oxidation colours

Permanent colour changes the natural colour of hair. When tiny colour molecules are mixed with hydrogen peroxide the colour penetrates the cuticle and is absorbed into the cortex. Here oxidation takes place causing the molecules to expand so the new colour remains permanently fixed within the hair. Permanent colours can lighten and colour, or darken and colour, natural hair in one application. The most usual forms of this type of colour are cream, gel or liquid.

- Manipulation of natural colour pigments.
- Small colour molecules penetrate the cuticle and enter the cortex.
- They develop into large molecules and remain fixed inside the cortex.
- Make the colour permanent.
- This chemical reaction is known as polymerisation.

Quasi-permanent colour

Quasi-permanent colours last for four to six weeks, gradually fading from the hair. They are ideal for refreshing tints, correcting colour, masking grey hair and adding fashion effects. They have the gentleness of a semi-permanent colour and the longevity of a permanent colour which fades out. Quasi-permanent colours will leave a slight regrowth depending on how often this product is used.

Chemistry of quasi-permanent colour

- Small- and medium-sized colour molecules.
- Para dye mixed with low volume developers.
- Cuticle gently swells to allow colour to penetrate into the cortex.
- Colour molecules gradually fade out.

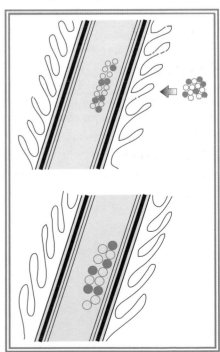

Figure 17.8 Action of permanent hair colour

High lift permanent colours

- Small colour molecules.
- Mixed with hydrogen peroxide.
- When mixed the molecule expands and gets trapped in the cortex.
- Usually lifts the colour for approximately 30 minutes.
- Deposits tone for the last 15 minutes.
- Can lift up to four shades depending on the volume peroxide used.

Faults and corrections

FAULTS	POSSIBLE CAUSES	CORRECTION
Patchy results	<ul><li>Insufficient product applied</li><li>Incorrect colour product mixing</li><li>Section too large</li><li>Overlapping previous colour</li><li>Re-growth too long</li></ul>	<ul><li>Reapply colour as required</li><li>Cleanse dark areas</li><li>Apply colour for long re-growth application</li></ul>
Scalp irritation	<ul><li>Peroxide too strong</li><li>Client allergic to tint</li><li>Hair washed immediately before colour application</li><li>Client scalp hot/perspiration</li><li>Colour not allowed to stand prior to colouring</li><li>Allergic reaction</li></ul>	<ul><li>Remove immediately with cool water</li><li>Do not wash the hair immediately prior to permanent colouring</li><li>Treat the hair and scalp gently. Colour may need to be removed</li><li>Ensure colour is allowed to stand</li><li>Always seek medical advice</li></ul>
Colour result too light	<ul><li>Re-confirm colour choice is correct</li><li>Cream developer used is too high</li></ul>	<ul><li>Reapply colour as required</li><li>Re-colour if shade difference is more than two levels</li></ul>
Colour too dark	<ul><li>Confirm colour choice is correct</li><li>Cream developer used is too low</li><li>Possible ash tone on hair</li></ul>	<ul><li>Cleanse colour to lighten</li><li>Use correct colour developer</li><li>Take ash tone into consideration and neutralise with corrective tone</li></ul>
Rapid colour fade	<ul><li>Insufficient development time</li><li>Cream developer too high</li><li>Undercoat too pale for shade applied</li><li>9% used on lengths and ends</li></ul>	<ul><li>Reapply colour for full development time</li><li>Use correct developer next time</li><li>Pre-colour before re-colouring</li><li>Re-mix colour with lower cream developer</li></ul>
Final result too red	<ul><li>Undercoat not considered. Natural warmth showing through</li><li>Insufficient development time</li></ul>	<ul><li>Choose a lighter target shade to avoid warmth from natural base</li><li>Leave on for full development time</li></ul>
Poor coverage	<ul><li>Insufficient product applied</li><li>Incorrect colour product mix</li><li>Sections too large</li><li>Resistant white hair</li></ul>	<ul><li>Re-apply colour as required</li><li>Mix correct colour</li><li>Re-apply to areas not covered</li><li>Pre-soften white hair and reapply</li></ul>

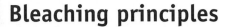

Bleaching principles

Levels of lightening

As the hair lightens the pigments are moved with the granular pigments dissolving first, leaving behind the diffuse pigment, which cannot be totally removed from the hair without destroying the hair fibre itself. The stages of this lightening process are called undercoats and correspond to a depth of colour.

Undercoat	Corresponding Depth
Red	1–5
Orange red	6
Orange	7
Yellow orange	8
Yellow	9
Pale Yellow	10

Types of bleaches

Cream bleach applications	Easy to apply Gives 1–5 shades lift	Good for scalp and full head
Oil bleach applications	Easy to apply Gives 1–3 shades lift	Good for scalp and full head
Emulsion bleach applications	Easy to apply Gives 1–5 shades lift	Good for scalp and full head
Powder bleach	Gives 1–5 shades lift	Good for highlighting. Can apply to scalp
Dust free bleach	Gives 1–5 shades lift	Good for highlighting. Can apply to scalp

- Bleach is a chemical used to lighten the colour of hair. To activate bleach, oxygen needs to be added. This is done by adding hydrogen peroxide.
- Once mixed and applied to the hair, the cuticle lifts allowing the bleach to penetrate.
- Oxygen is released from the peroxide and reacts with the natural hair pigments, making them colourless.
- As the bleach works the hair will gradually lighten.
- Dark brown will lighten through red, orange and yellow. A violet-based toner must then be added to neutralise the yellow tones.
- Very light brown hair to blonde hair will go very pale yellow and may not need a toner.
- Over bleaching will destroy the structure of the hair. This can be due to:

  ▷ using peroxide that is too strong

  ▷ processing the hair for too long

  ▷ overlapping

▸ combing the bleach through the hair

▸ bleaching hair in poor condition.

● To avoid over-bleaching always test a cutting of the hair prior to application.

Hydrogen peroxide

Hydrogen peroxide comes in liquid or cream form. It is described in volume and percentage strength. The volume strength refers to the amount of oxygen that is produced, i.e.

● 1 litre of 30 volume would produce 30 litres of oxygen, leaving 1 litre of water.

● The percentage strength indicates how much of the solution is actually peroxide, the rest being water, i.e. 100 grammes of 9% would mean 9% is peroxide and the remaining 91% is water

10 volume = 3% 30 volume = 9%

20 volume = 6% 40 volume = 12%

Faults and corrections

Faults	Possible causes	Correction
Uneven colour result	● Poor application ● Product consistency too thick	● Take fine sections ● Re-apply bleach as necessary
Scalp irritation	● Peroxide too strong ● Client allergic to tint	● Remove immediately with cool water
Hair breakage	● Over-porous ● Over-processed ● Overlapping ● Combed through too much ● Incorrect selection of colour	● Remove immediately ● Cut if possible ● Use restructurant/deep penetrating conditioner
Result too yellow	● Under-processed ● Base too dark ● Incorrect selection of product	● Do a porosity test – if OK re-bleach
Seepage of product	● Incorrect application of materials and product ● Too much product applied ● Incorrect mixing of product	● Spot colour areas too light
Bands of yellow	● Too long between application ● Different strengths of developer used ● Different development time followed	● Lighten hair root application every four weeks ● Check recommended instructions for use ● Check previous application record card
Toner after bleaching not taking at root	● Undercoat lightened too much ● Lengths and ends sensitised, grabbing toner appearing heavy	● Pre-colour root area ● Cleanse lengths and ends
Toner washes out too quickly	● Undercoat lightened too high ● Poor condition ● Insufficient development time	● Reassess condition; apply slightly darker shade ● Pre-colour before re-applying toner ● Follow recommended development time

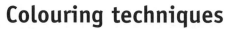

Colouring techniques

There are so many techniques available that hairdressers nowadays are spoilt for choice. Colouring is one of the most exciting areas. Stylists can really get creative making hair look anything from natural to avant-garde. These are just some of the techniques available to you:

Technique	Method	Result
Highlights/lowlights Weave out sections of hair	● Cap ● Foil ● Meche ● Freehand ● Spatula ● Colour pens ● Frosting ● Tipping	● Short hair, textured effect ● Fine or thick sections; all hair lengths; shiny, subtle, fashionable, partial head or full head applications gives texture or overall colour enhancement ● Same as foil ● Good on short, spiky hair or single lights or lowlights ● Good for low lighting on all hair lengths ● Good for colouring hair lines and adding colour ● Good on short hair, lightening all the ends ● Good for colouring woven tips or cap method by just applying to ends of the hair
Block colouring Colouring a whole section opposite to weaves	● Underlighting ● Down lighting ● Partial application ● Tip application	● Suitable on all hair lengths to the front and crown areas to add colour and shine ● To give depth in specified areas to give three-dimensional effects to enhance the haircut ● To add colour exactly where required to enhance the haircut ● Good on short to medium length hair to give texture and add colour
Colour effects	● Polishing ● Tortoiseshell ● Sponge on ● Texture ● Conditioning ● Marbling ● Painting ● Stencilling ● Herringbone	● 1–2 shades lighter to give shine. Good on bobs and solid haircuts ● To give texture ● To create tones that merge into one another. Good on reds and coppers ● To create fine, medium and coarse textures to enhance the haircut ● To give shine and a healthy glow ● Creative colouring technique; good on medium and long one-length hair ● Colour any shape or form to accentuate haircut ● To replicate images. Good on clipper haircuts ● Used subtly, can make hair look natural depending on how many colours are used. Two to three colours, various shades of blonde, or one light colour and one dark colour, or various reds and coppers in a herringbone effect
Creative colour	● Effect depending on tools used	● Packaging e.g. bubble wrap, polystyrene packaging applied to hair and colouring in between
Full head applications	● All over colour	● Good on any length to go lighter or darker ● Good for colouring white hair ● Good for complete colour change
Two-tone applications	● Hairline perimeter section ● Innerline section	● Perimeter darker can reverse result. Depends on section thickness ● Inner area lighter can reverse result. Depends on section thickness

UNIT H32 CONTRIBUTE TO THE PLANNING AND IMPLEMENTATION OF PROMOTIONAL ACTIVITIES

18

1 Contribute to the planning and preparation of promotional activities

2 Implement promotional activities

3 Participate in the evaluation of promotional activities

CHAPTER CONTENTS

- *Salon Promotion*
- *Planning the Promotional Activity*
- *Characteristics of Differing Promotional Opportunities*

- *Summary*
- *Further Development Activities*
- *Review Questions*
- *Additional information*

Salon promotion

Any feature or activity that attracts the attention of the client or potential client to the salon can be said to be promotional. In most cases positive features and activities have the best effect. It was Brendan Behan who said 'There's no such thing as bad publicity', but for hairdressing salons some adverse publicity can inhibit clients from visiting the salon.

Promotion may take the form of projecting an image or range of services through:

- staff team appearance
- salon window display
- advertising
- distribution of information
- direct marketing
- demonstration
- fashion shows
- publicity stunts
- charity promotions.

Planning the promotional activity

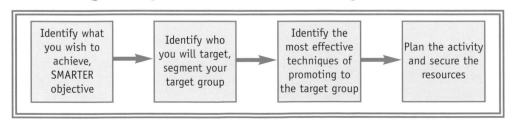

| Identify what you wish to achieve, SMARTER objective | → | Identify who you will target, segment your target group | → | Identify the most effective techniques of promoting to the target group | → | Plan the activity and secure the resources |

Figure 18.2 Planning a promotional activity

Figure 18.1 A promotional stand

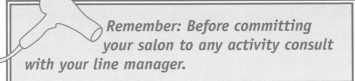

Identify what you wish to achieve

For all forms of promotional activity be clear about why it is being undertaken and what you wish to achieve. This may be discussed initially with your line manager and success criteria or performance measures agreed. These performance measures are best stated as SMARTER objectives as they will steer you towards achieving exactly what is required – see Chapter 5 for more information about setting SMARTER targets. It is likely that the objectives for promotional activity will be linked to increases in:

> *Remember: Before committing your salon to any activity consult with your line manager.*

> *Remember: SMARTER – Specific, Measurable, Achievable, Relevant, Time Bound, Evaluated and Resourced.*

- client numbers
- specified groups of clients
- sales or salon takings
- specific treatments.

Identify who you will target

Be quite clear about the groups you are targeting. This may be determined by your line manager or left for you and your team to decide. Segmenting in this context is a process of grouping people together by particular characteristics. You may have segmented your target group by one or more of the following:

- Gender – male or female.
- Age – grouping into age ranges.
- Ethnic or cultural groups.
- Income groups.
- Work roles.
- Where people live.
- Places they visit.

You must be satisfied there are sufficient people within the target group to satisfy the objectives you have agreed, and certain that the target group has a direct link to the objectives that have been set.

Example A

Your objective is to increase the number of clients who have hair colour in the salon during weekday afternoons throughout the autumn by 50%. Your segmentation may identify:

- Gender, female – more likely to be available during afternoons in non-holiday periods.
- Age range 35 to 50 – more likely not to have children to collect from school.
- Income group – upper and middle class – available surplus income.
- Work role – non-working, therefore available in the afternoons.

Example B

Alternatively, if your objective is to introduce 75 new teenage clients for haircutting to the salon during the July period, your segmentation may identify:

- Gender – either male or female.
- Age range – 16 to 18 years.

- Work role – just completed examinations at school.
- Where people live – within a set distance from a local school with a sixth form.
- Places they visit – local sports centre, shopping mall, youth club.

You may decide that the objectives of a particular promotional activity are relevant to all groups of people. This provides a very wide potential target group of people but it may make it more difficult to focus the promotional activity to meet everyone's expectations.

Identifying relevant promotional activities

Having identified who you are targeting with your promotion, you may then consider the range of promotional opportunities available to you that are relevant to the target group. You will need to consider:

- What activity or activities are likely to attract or interest the target group.
- When to implement the activity most effectively.
- How to inform the target group most effectively.
- What the likely costs are and what budget, if any, you have available.

Including your staff team and line manager in these activities will add to the resource of ideas and will encourage participation. Undertake field research talking to people from the identified target group, and gather their ideas and thoughts about what activity would most attract them. The more people you talk to, the more likely you are to determine promotional activities that will widely appeal to your target group. Talk to people who have previously undertaken promotions, find out what worked well for them, what did not work well and what advice they would give you. It is most likely that the final decision will rest with the salon owner, and you may need to discuss your ideas with either your line manager or the salon owner before final decisions are made and planning started.

Planning promotional activities

It is unlikely that you will undertake your promotional activity in isolation. Involve others who can bring support and expertise to the team. Promotional activities provide a good opportunity to develop teamwork and spirit within the salon. You may already have some clear ideas yourself or have been given a clear directive about the format that the promotional activity will take by your line manager.

Effective communication within the promotion team and a clear understanding of what is expected of each team member both in general and for specific actions, is essential. It is often best to start by having a meeting with the whole team where the objectives of the promotion are explained and ideas for the promotion activity are described. Guide and encourage team members to contribute ideas for the promotional activity. Each idea should be reviewed for its appropriateness and a decision made.

Identify each task that must be undertaken and decide a logical sequence in which these actions should be taken. Some actions occur consecutively and others occur concurrently.

If there is a predetermined date when the promotion is to occur, you may wish to work backwards from the event to set target dates by which key stages of the preparation must be undertaken.

> *Remember: Consecutive tasks take place one after the other; concurrent tasks may occur at the same time or overlap.*

A process of planning will involve:

- being clear about the objectives and required outcomes of the promotion
- identifying the date by which the promotion must occur
- listing all tasks that have to be undertaken, no matter how simple

- grouping the tasks into a sequential order, identifying date for completion, and drawing upon previous experiences if available

- agreeing an allocation of tasks to individuals or teams, drawing on the expertise or contacts of individuals

- agreeing dates to review progress

- allowing time for slippage or handling unexpected events

- being prepared to respond to changes in plans if required.

Ensure that you have sufficient helpers for the preparation and for the promotional event itself.

Schedule time to evaluate the effectiveness of the promotion and to share experiences.

> *Remember: When planning your promotion do your homework – find out if any other events will clash with yours or if there are events that you could work with.*

It is very likely that your promotion event will use more than one promotional opportunity. For example, you may be planning to promote your salon by providing a demonstration of hair fashions. It is very likely that you will encourage your staff team to talk about it to their clients, advertise the event within the salon and other local shops, contact local relevant groups, produce a press release and send this to your local newspaper and radio, and distribute information leaflets or tickets. You should plan for these activities and schedule them so that they build information and sustain local interest up to the event. Allow sufficient time for printing of tickets, etc.

Characteristics of differing promotional opportunities

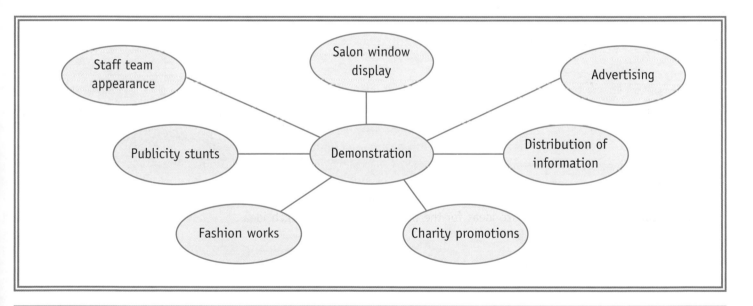

Figure 18.3 Promotional opportunities

Staff team appearance

This should be considered an on-going promotional opportunity. The way your salon staff appear and act projects a message to your clients. This promotional opportunity may be used to influence both existing and prospective clients.

- Staff hairstyles can be used as a living style book giving indications to clients of the style of hairdressing you provide, the range of services you offer and the quality of your work. Staff hair can show how colour can enhance a fashion look or demonstrate a current look that you are promoting.

- Staff dress can project an image of the salon that will often relate to a particular segment of the population. Your salon may already have a corporate image, one that applies to all salon activities, and that will have been planned to relate to a particular segment or to maintain a particular image. Styles of dress can relate to particular people and can provide indications or build expectations of the style of hairdressing undertaken. It is very likely that a prospective client will assume that a hairstylist whose own hair and style of dress is very avant-garde will provide similar hairstyling. This can sometimes impart confusing or incorrect messages.

- Styles of language will often relate to particular client groups. People using similar styles of language or vocabulary will relate more readily to the salon's staff.

If your salon does not currently have a corporate approach to the way staff appear, you may wish to consider this opportunity.

Remember: Many local authorities have legal requirements – bye laws – relating to the use of protective clothing in the salon. Information may be obtained from your local town hall.

Salon window display

The salon façade and window display provides an opportunity for continuous promotion to potential and existing clients who pass by. Messages about the salon are conveyed by the style of frontage. It may appear very modern and functional, conveying a message of prompt, cost effective but quality services. It may appear classical and luxurious, conveying a message of high cost and luxurious service. You may wish to consult with professional builders who specialise in shop fitments for advice. You can often obtain information about these in your local telephone directory, features and advertisements in the hairdressing trade press and by asking other salon owners who they have used to provide this service It is very likely that decisions regarding the exterior of the salon frontage will be made by the proprietor and/or salon manager. Your contributions may be requested.

The actual salon window provides a continuous promotional opportunity. You may decide to provide a view of the salon interior, allowing the salon activity to promote itself. The salon window can provide the opportunity to display retail products or to promote your hairdressing through posters, pictures, etc. Your window display should always appear fresh and clean. Sunlight can cause colours to fade and products to react. You may get ideas by researching how other local salons use their window areas. Research nationally by reviewing hairdressing trade publications.

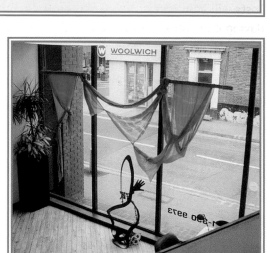

Figure 18.4 A salon window display

Advertising

Advertising may be used independently or linked to other promotional activities. Advertising will usually be local, as it would normally be unrealistic to expect clients to travel a great distance to visit your salon. Therefore to advertise your salon to a very wide geographic area would not be an effective use of financial resources. This may not be the case when your salon is located within a central area that people often travel considerable distances to get to, e.g. attracted by a retail complex.

Remember: Local planning regulations may restrict the options available for your salon frontage.

On a national level your advertising may be within:

- national consumer magazines
- consumer hairdressing directories

- national newspapers
- website.

On a local level your advertising may be within:

- local newspapers
- local telephone directories
- local television or radio
- direct mail shot to local individuals or groups
- local leaflet drop
- public transport advertising
- posters.

Costs will vary considerably between these forms of advertising. Initial enquiries should enable you to determine the costs. Having determined them, you should consider how each fits with your target group.

Newspapers

The following information is usually available from the newspaper's advertising department:

- target readership
- how many newspapers are sold (distributed if a free paper)
- geographic areas to which the newspaper is distributed
- copy date – the deadline for material
- forthcoming advertising features with which you may link.

Unless you are using an advertisement consisting of words only, there may be additional costs incurred for any drawings or artwork. By using a personal computer you may be able to produce your own artwork, or link with a hairdressing manufacturer or wholesaler who has templates for general use and who may share the costs. Remember to check the accuracy of any wording and dates included in your advert carefully before approving it for publication.

Advertising within newspapers will often be more effective if it is built into an editorial feature. When planning your promotion consider how you can gain the interest of your local newspaper. The newspaper will be most interested in writing if the promotion has:

- local interest – it includes or impacts on local people
- an unusual story
- celebrity involvement
- charity involvement/support
- photographic opportunity – to gain maximum impact you will need to arrange this to occur before the event
- consumer information – a new and interesting product or service, a unique process.

Build these features into your press release. Keep it short and to the point and always include what it is about, the salon name, the location, the uniqueness of the event, dates and content, and who to contact for more information. Find out, by telephoning the newspaper, where to send the press release. Have available any further information, background and reasons for the event and the people involved, history of the salon, clientele, and relevant photo opportunities.

If your promotion has more than a local interest you may be able to gain attention from a national newspaper or consumer magazine. Gaining support and linking with a manufacturer that advertises within the magazine can help when attempting to gain the editor's interest.

Editorials

Editorials are great as you do not have to pay to advertise, yet you inform readers of any news interests. So you need to keep them interesting and ensure you get your news over in a way that can be beneficial to you as a salon/organisation. Below is a sample script of 150 words. It is a good idea to keep a selection of quality photographs as you never know when you might need them. It is better to use slides or negatives but check with the newspapers as to which format they prefer. Sometimes the quality of digitalised photographs may not be suitable.

'Submitting photographs of your hairdressing to consumer hairstyle guide magazines can be an effective way of promoting the salon. Contact the magazine to confirm the format in which they will accept photographs for publication, the information and permissions they require, to whom to send the photographs, and their deadline date.

Local radio and television

This type of advertising is usually more costly than newspaper advertising, and the cost of preparing the advertisement is generally too high to use for a one-off event. However, as with newspapers, newsworthy events can often gain a level of editorial coverage. The greatest level of publicity is frequently gained from the media following the event, when more material is available. The effectiveness of this form of promotion will, in part, depend upon the target group and whether they watch or listen to locally provided services.

Remember: It is likely that you will have very little control on how your event is reported and presented.

As with newspapers, if you plan to access local radio or television you should produce a press release. Be prepared to provide further information and to be interviewed as part of the production. Find out when the production team are due to arrive at your event and plan to provide them with interview and photographic opportunities as soon as possible. In most cases their time is very limited. Television crews will often focus on visually sensational shots and can be disruptive to the event in their efforts to get the best camera angles and sound levels. Generally, the promotional impact of these will be almost immediate, provided that no

Remember: You will have more control over the content of paid advertising than the content of an editorial. The credibility of editorial material is much greater with the public. Prepare what you wish to say when following up a press release.

"Kingston College hairdressing students were privileged to watch top stylists from London and Korea at work when they recently visited Kingston College. As part of a programme designed to bring the best training to students, Michael Razo, Dino Karvelis and Seshi Park gave an inspiring insight into the art of hair styling. These gifted hairdressers demonstrated current fashion looks on models of all ages to demonstrate how good technique, styling and finishing is essential when students graduate and go into employment."

"The hairdressers are part of a team who will be delivering hairdressing training on the internet through the International Beauty College (IBC), of which Kingston College forms a part. Students joining the IBC scheme will eventually be able to access training through the internet at home, while further training and assessment at Kingston College will enable them to gain qualifications at all levels to assist them in their chosen career."

major news stories occur. If this is the case it may be very likely that your event will never be broadcast. Often copies of a television recording can be purchased from the company and used to further promote the salon.

Distribution of information

Direct marketing is targeting promotional information directly to identified people or groups. This is a frequently used promotion technique and has the advantage over blanket advertising in that the identification of those being targeted is known and their responses can be monitored. You will need the contact information of your target group. Your salon may already hold this information within its client records.

If the people you wish to promote to are not included within your current client database you will need to gain access to further data. If you need to contact a limited number of people directly, e.g. local council dignitaries, you may be able to create your own database by telephoning the council offices and requesting names, titles and contact addresses. You can also obtain information through the electoral role that is available at the post office or local public library and via a range of internet sites.

> Remember: The information your salon holds about its clients is subject to the Data Protection Act and its use is controlled, see Chapter 3. Check with your line manager before using this information for promotional purposes.

If you wish to target the individual membership of a local group directly you may find that you can achieve this most effectively by providing the group secretary with the appropriate information in pre-stamped envelopes. They can then be addressed by him or her and will not require personal information to be provided to you. Your local public library will often have a list of local groups and societies, together with points of contact.

Direct marketing can enable you to send named invitations for promotional events directly to the individual, and to be able to confirm their acceptance by telephone. This can be useful when planning seating and refreshments.

Local leaflet drops

Printed information can be distributed to households within a specified geographic area. This form of promotion enables you to target people who live within a small area. Any leaflets distributed in this way must be interesting and grab the recipient's attention immediately. With the high volume of unsolicited mail sent to households today there is a tendency to throw this type of material in the rubbish bin without reading it fully. Including a free competition on the front of these leaflets can encourage people to read and respond.

Providing a small reward for those who follow up these promotion leaflets can help you to monitor their success. It can help you determine the appropriateness of this method when planning future promotions.

Demonstrations

You may decide to provide a demonstration to clients and/or potential clients. The exact nature of your demonstration will vary according to your objectives. If you are promoting a particular product or service the demonstration will most probably centre around this, its features and benefits. If the objective is broader, possibly to attract a particular target group, it may need to be more responsive to the particular needs of those watching. Having identified the objectives and your audience, you will need to decide where best to undertake this. You may ask yourself:

● Should the salon go to the audience or will they come to the salon?

● What type of location will the target group wish to visit?

● At what time and day of the week will the target group attend?

● Will the demonstration be a single timed event with a single audience or a continuous loop with an audience that comes and goes?

● What will attract the target group?

- What specialist equipment will be required?
- What is the budget, if any?

Venue

The answers to these questions may guide you when determining an appropriate location for your demonstration. Some locations will charge a fee for use; others may not do so if there are benefits either the venue or its visitors will accrue. You may be able to gain financial sponsorship from manufacturers or wholesalers that your salon purchases from. If they are unable to provide direct financial support, they may be able to support you by providing products for use free of charge, samples to give to the audience or help in marketing the event. Of course, they will wish to gain public recognition for their contribution. Discuss this with your sales representatives.

To attract busy people during normal shopping hours you may find demonstrating within the concourse of a shopping mall most effective. Undertake research to confirm who visits the mall, the day of the week and time of day to gain maximum audience numbers and suitable locations within the mall. Research the management of the mall and who you should contact in order to pursue this. It is likely that your demonstration, while a continuous loop, will provide impact within short timescales as the audience will usually be transient and lose interest very quickly. Owing to the changing audience, it may be most appropriate to repeat the same demonstration over and over again.

> *Remember: It is often more effective for the salon to go to the target group than the group to come to the salon.*

If your objective relates to a target group that already congregates, research the possibilities of accessing this meeting for your demonstration. If the target group are members of a club or association you may be able to provide your demonstration as part of a group meeting at their meeting place. Some groups may favour visiting the salon. Research your local groups, talk to their secretaries to identify where they meet, the frequency of their meetings and the membership profile. Other target groups may congregate but are not actually members of a club that has specified club meetings. Research these locations, those who usually attend and what opportunities there may be to provide a demonstration. Locations may include schools, discos and sports centres. Most of these venues have duty managers who will be able to provide an initial response to your enquiry and proposals.

If you decide that you will hire a demonstration venue, research those that are suitable. Consider:

> *Remember: Most people will not give their time to attend or give their attention to something that holds little interest to them. Identify the key feature that will create and hold an interest for the target group.*

- Location – will and can your target group travel to the venue easily?

- Style – does the ambiance of the venue fit your target group?

- Facilities – if required, are there adequate facilities for audience refreshments, seating, preparation, staging, lighting, electricity for equipment and heating?

- Size – is the venue large enough or too large for your event?

- Cost – is it within your budget?

Hotels often have rooms for hire that range in size and are usually able to provide the facilities required. You should also consider the use of sports centres, community and civic centres, village and church halls, club and society halls, and schools. Many of these will hire rooms and to varying degrees will have a range of facilities appropriate to your demonstration's needs.

When demonstrating to people who normally visit your salon, provided there is adequate room and facilities, the salon can be used as a suitable location. Out of normal opening hours the salon often provides the ideal location. If your salon is located within a department store or shopping mall, there may be restrictions to operating times due to the closure of the entire building. Within the salon, tools, equipment and preparation facilities are usually available. Demonstrations that take place in the salon during normal opening times can be effective as often there is an audience created by clients visiting the salon for their hair appointments. Care must be taken not to have a detrimental impact on the business by taking staff away from normal productive working, or using floor space that creates an unsafe situation or prevents the salon from functioning normally. Any event should be discussed with your line manager beforehand and the likely impacts considered.

> **Remember:** When you have confirmed the budget for the demonstration maintain a list of all planned expenditure and keep within the agreed level. If you identify the need to exceed the budget discuss this with your line manager beforehand, having identified the exact level of budget required and any source.

Demonstration format

While identifying the appropriate venue you will also need to plan the demonstration. The format may be guided by the venue itself. For example, it is unlikely that your audience will be seated if you are demonstrating in a shopping mall concourse. A theatre-style venue can restrict interaction between the demonstrators and their audience. It is best if the audience is encouraged to ask questions about what is being demonstrated as this provides you with greater promotional opportunities, as well as satisfying their need and keeping people's attention.

If the demonstration is a timed event that has a definite beginning and end, you should plan and rehearse each stage:

- Opening – how you plan to gain people's attention and introduce yourselves to the audience. Open with impact.
- Set the scene – how you will explain what the audience will see and what they will gain from this.
- Demonstration – how you will demonstrate, project the key messages to the audience, involve the audience, and maintain interest.
- Closure – how you will ensure that the audience knows what they should do next to access the services of the salon, summarise the key messages you wish to project and close with impact.

At this stage identify all of the equipment that you will need. Do not assume that equipment will be available – check and confirm it with those responsible. If you plan to have a raised stage, confirm its dimensions so that you can rehearse on a similar sized space. Rehearse how people will enter and leave the stage or demonstration area. Consider when and how this will be constructed and arrange for this to take place.

Lighting

Look at lighting. You may just require general bright light; check that this is available and is sufficiently bright to see the detail of your demonstration. If you require specialist lighting, follow spots for example, make arrangements well in advance. Plan and rehearse this and any cues for lighting changes or effects. If you are using background music throughout your demonstration this should also be identified. Choose the music you wish and ensure that it is in the correct format for the available sound equipment. Have a back-up version available in case of failure. Unless you plan to maintain the same music level (volume) throughout your demonstration you will need someone to adjust this on cue. Plan and rehearse this. If you are using a microphone, practise with this to work out correct sound levels and ensure that it is held or located close enough to the person speaking to be audible and so that the person is able to continue working, if required. For small audiences

> **Remember:** For safety, always us a qualified expert to configure any lighting, sound and stage electrical fitments.

> **Remember:** When rehearsing in an empty room the volume will sound louder than when it is full of people.

your own voice may project. Remember, however, that when there are levels of ambient noise your voice may not project so well. You may be able to gain the assistance of an enthusiast from your local amateur dramatics society to provide expertise in lighting and sound. When using some venues you may be restricted to using only their technicians.

Equipment and accessories

Often you will find that other organisations are willing to loan equipment, clothing, etc, for events, particularly if they are charity related. Ensure that anything loaned to you is adequately insured against loss or damage and that arrangements have been made for their collection, safe storage and prompt return. Often organisations loaning these items will appreciate recognition of this during the event and in any publicity material that you issue. If you are looking for an interesting diversion during your presentation, you might consider linking with a local fashion store to provide a fashion show or to an amateur dance group to provide a presentation. Effective liaison with other participating organisations is essential to ensure a seamless presentation.

Identify what equipment will be required to be set in place for the demonstration, how this will occur and who will be responsible. If equipment is to be moved during the demonstration confirm how this will occur, who will do it and how the cue for this will be given. Make a checklist of all resources that you will require and confirm who will be responsible for ensuring each is available at the appropriate time. Confirm any additional costs that are likely to be incurred and incorporate these into your budget. If the required resources exceed your budget, you may have to decide which are essential for the success of the demonstration and which may be disregarded. Ensure that relevant people are informed of changes in resource requirements.

Even for those who are experienced in demonstrating, planning and practice is essential. All of those involved both in front of and behind the scenes should be fully conversant with their role and responsibilities, and how their roles relate to those of others. It will be most supportive to those who have not previously demonstrated or worked in front of an audience to rehearse this to develop confidence.

Script

Produce a script for the demonstration that indicates the:

- sequence of events – key prompts or cue for action or changes, what will occur, who will be involved, equipment that is needed either to be set out beforehand or carried on during the demonstration

- timing for each action

- music, lighting or any special effects if required, with their cues for start and end.

Having practised with the script you may need to make adjustments to make it practicable. Adjustments may be to timings or activities, positioning of people on stage, cues for changes and allocation of responsibilities. Ensure that all of those involved in the demonstration are included in the rehearsal. By doing this you will be certain that everyone is aware of their role, they are not overloaded and are able to undertake each of the tasks allocated. Do not be afraid to make adjustments, but when finalised ensure that those who need it have a copy of the final version and that they work to it.

Remember: When rehearsing, encourage helpers to act and respond as an audience as this will support those who are very nervous on stage.

Remember: For demonstrations where you encourage your audience to participate by watching very closely or trying a technique themselves, consider the benefits of not using a raised stage so that there are fewer barriers to this involvement.

Remember: If you are heavily committed to providing the demonstration you may benefit from delegating the responsibility for co-ordinating the overall event on the day so that you can concentrate on your own role.

Schedule

When you are satisfied with your presentation and how it will take place, finalise the sequence of events, produce a schedule and ensure that all are aware of these plans. Include within this schedule adequate time for preparation, time for late arrivals or travel difficulties. Be realistic with your plans.

The demonstration

Just before the start of the demonstration the co-ordinator should check that everyone is in place and ready to proceed. They should check that the demonstration team is ready and will have the final decision about when the demonstration starts. It may be appropriate to defer the start of a demonstration if not all of the audience is present. However, balance any such decision with the feelings of frustration of the audience who are present may experience and the impact on the time of completion this may have.

Remember that people have limited attention spans so your demonstration must be short, interesting and varied. Most members of the public find technical information useful but not necessarily interesting. They are often more interested in seeing the end product with a limited insight into how it is achieved. Prepare completed models to introduce to the audience during lengthy technical demonstrations, arrange for part of the work to be undertaken prior to the demonstration or out of sight while other aspects are being introduced. Use models that your target group can relate to, for example, when demonstrating to a teenage group use teenage models, when demonstrating to a more mature group use models who are similar in age, and when demonstrating to a target group who are of mixed ages use a variety of models. People will often associate better with the content of the demonstration if a model is drawn from one of their group.

If the audience is to leave with a particular message or information, produce a brief fact sheet. This will help to avoid confused messages or missed opportunities. The sheet can provide a point of contact, details of how to follow up and enquiries. To gain further audience interaction, to obtain people's feedback on the demonstration and to develop a database of details and preferences, use a questionnaire that can easily be completed at the time. Provide pens or pencils, and consider encouraging their completion with a free entry to a prize draw. This can provide further promotional opportunities.

Fashion shows

You may be asked to undertake hairstyling for the models of a fashion show being held by a local store. Discuss this with your line manager before committing the salon to this joint enterprise.

> *Remember: Following a demonstration there will be a need to dismantle, remove and return equipment used. Make arrangements for this to be undertaken. Often a delay in this can result in increased rental costs.*

To support you in preparing for this, research and consider:

- the type and style of clothes that will be shown – the image to be projected
- the people who will be modelling the clothes
- the time available for the preparation of the hair – the number of styles and the frequency of changes, if any
- the facilities available to prepare the hair – adequate lighting, electrical supplies, water supplies, materials to be used.

You may be restricted in what can be done to the models' hair due to the available budget for consumables, the models' wishes and the preparation time available. Undertake as much preparation beforehand as possible.

Ensure before the event that all models are aware of the time they should be available for their hair preparation, and in what state their hair should be in when they arrive. Allocate sufficient time for all the hairdressing to be

> *Remember: The use of added hair can be an effective strategy for rapidly changing the models' image.*

undertaken within the planned schedule. Allow additional time to be able to cope with unforeseen situations, for example late arrival or changes in hairstyles.

Publicity stunts

Publicity can take many forms and attract attention to the salon or to a planned event. Publicity is usually associated with the presence of the media to aid the publicity impact. Effective publicity events have considerable visual impact and create public interest. These events can include:

> *Remember: Incorporating a clothes fashion presentation into a hairdressing demonstration will provide an additional element of interest for the audience.*

- producing extreme hairstyle effects, often that link to a current local or national theme or event
- undertaking a task in extreme conditions or setting a record often linked to a number of actions that can be completed within a specified time. This is often associated with sponsorship.

In order to gain maximum publicity, inform the media of the event in sufficient time giving details of the content, when and where it will take place, its objectives, and who will be involved. If a charity is involved, give details of this also. This information can be presented in the form of a press release as described earlier in this section. To gain most visual impact within the media, ensure there are sufficient photo opportunities.

> *Remember: A publicity stunt that is kept secret will have no benefit. At the appropriate time ensure that people are aware of the event.*

Careful planning is essential to bring all the elements of the publicity stunt together at the correct time. Communicate your plans to the team, allocate roles and responsibilities. Check that what should occur does occur. Do not leave things to chance. Remind people of the event and confirm their intention to attend or participate. You may only have one chance to gain publicity from this event so make the most of the opportunity.

Often publicity stunts can attract more media coverage if they are linked with fund raising for charity.

Charity promotions

Raising funds for charity can provide good promotional opportunities for your salon while at the same time supporting a worthy cause. Most people are willing to support a charitable cause either by their attendance, participation before or during the event, or by providing materials to help.

Charity events may take the form of a specific hairdressing event to raise funds so that both the salon and the charity have a high profile within the event, or in the form of staff participation in a charity event, such as a fun run, where the charity has a high profile and the salon gains promotion through its involvement.

Following all promotional activities, evaluate the effectiveness of the activity and how it has supported the achievement of its objectives. Make notes to remind you of the aspects that worked well, as well as those that were less effective and use this information to guide you when planning any future event.

Summary

The promotion of the salon as a business may occur in a variety of ways. There is a need to continuously promote the appropriate image of the salon as well as undertaking one-off promotions with a particular focus. A programme of continuous one-off promotions will maintain the salon's profile in the community.

You have been given an overview of diverse ways this can be achieved so that you can effectively contribute to planning and implementing such actions. The suggestions provided within this section are not exhaustive and you should remain receptive to new ideas and suggestions.

Further development activities

Research opportunities to undertake a promotional activity for the salon. Identify what you would wish to achieve for the salon and consider the range of promotional activities that will enable you to achieve these SMARTER objectives. Create a plan for how this promotional activity would take place, the target group, who it may involve, what physical resources would be required, the budget required and how the success of the promotion would be measured. Discuss your idea with your line manager and gain their agreement before committing yourself or your salon to any actions.

Review Questions

1. State two benefits for the salon in promoting activities.

2. State four ways that you may segment target groups for promotion.

3. State six types of promotional activity that are relevant to promoting hairdressing.

4. How can staff appearance influence the perceptions of your clients?

Additional information

Useful websites

Website Addresses	Content
www.habia.org.uk	Hairdressing and Beauty Industry Authority. Downloads available including references to other websites
www.bbc-safety.co.uk	Free advice on health and safety
www.haircouncil.org.uk	UK statutory body for hairdressing
www.lookfantastic.com	Professional hairdressing products and advice
www.laurandp.co.uk	Educational publications for development of professional hairdressing
www.scott999.fsnet.co.uk	Hairdressing product information
www.nexus.com	Range of hairdressing products
www.tigi.co.uk	Range of hairdressing products
www.schwarzkopf.com	Range of hairdressing products
www.loreal.com	Range of hairdressing products

Magazines and journals

- *Hairdressers Journal*
- *Creative Head*
- *Estetica/Cutting Edge*
- *Black Beauty and Hair*

GLOSSARY

Current look Refers to styles that are currently fashionable.

Emerging look Refers to a commercial look that is the forerunner of fashion, i.e. next season's looks.

Enhancing the salon's image This phrase is used to convey that the final effect of look achieved is in line with that which the salon wishes to give to achieve its targeted position within the commercial market.

Factors influencing the service Anything that could affect the hairdressing service.

Fading This is a term often used in African-Caribbean barbering. It describes a form of tapering that goes into the haircut, possibly as far as the crown.

Fishtail plait (also known as a Herringbone plait) A four-strand plait achieved by crossing four pieces of hair over each other to create a 'herringbone' look.

Freehand The cutting of hair without holding it in place.

Fusing A method of attaching a micro-strand of added hair to the natural hair. Methods of fusing are using a heated appliance to melt synthetic hair or to melt polymer resin.

Goddess braiding These are extra-large cane rows consisting of two to five cane rows swept up on the top of the head.

Incompatibility This refers to chemicals that do not work together and may have an adverse reaction.

Legal requirements This refers to laws affecting the way businesses are operated, how the salon or workplace is set up and maintained, people in employment and the systems of working that must be maintained. Of particular importance are the COSHH Regulations, the Electricity at Work Regulations and the Cosmetic Products (Safety) Regulations.

Limits of own authority The extent of your responsibility as determined by your own job description and workplace policies.

Manufacturer's instructions Explicit guidance issued by manufacturers or suppliers of products or equipment, concerning their safe and efficient use.

Massage techniques
Effleurage A gentle, stroking movement.
Petrissage A slow, firm kneading movement.
Friction A vigorous rubbing movement using the finger pads. It is stimulating rather than relaxing and is not always carried out. It is only done for a few minutes, working from front to back.
Rotary A firm circular movement using the pads of the fingers over the surface of the scalp.

Moisturisers Products that add moisture to hair.

Outlines The perimeter of a haircut, beard, moustache or sideburn shape.

Personal presentation This includes` personal hygiene; use of personal protection equipment; clothing and accessories suitable to the particular workplace.

Personal Protective Equipment (PPE) You are required to use and wear the appropriate protective equipment or clothing during colouring, perming and relaxing services. Protective gloves and apron are the normal requirement for yourself.

Post-damping lotion Any product applied to wound hair (e.g. perming lotion).

Potentially Infectious condition A medical condition or state of health that may be transmitted to others.

Pre-damping lotions Any product applied to hair prior to winding (e.g. Booster, perming lotions, wrap humectants).

Pre-perm treatment A product that is applied to the hair prior to a chemical service to even out porosity along the hair shaft.

Pressing A technique that uses a thermal pressing comb to straighten the hair.

Quasi-permanent colour Colouring products that should be treated as permanent colours in terms of testing and future services.

Rearranger Ammonium-thiogycollate-based product used to pre-soften tight/curly hair prior to winding a perm.

Resources Anything used to aid the delivery and completion of the service (eg. towels, gowns, equipment, consumable items).

Restyle This refers to a significant change in either length, shape, style, volume or weight of the hair.

Rolls When dressing long hair, 'rolls' will also cover 'pleats'.

Salon requirements Any hairdressing procedures or work rules issued by the salon management.

Salon services Covers all the services offered in our workplace.

Scalp plaits These can also be known as a French Plait, a Cane Row or Corn Row Plait.

Sculpting This is the process of creating three-dimensional shapes within a haircut.

Sharps A term used by the Health and Safety Executive to describe sharp objects. In the context of hairdressing sharps include scissors, razors and razor blades which may have bye-laws covering their disposal.

Silky locks Locks created by wrapping the hair with added artificial hair down the length of the hair.

Slither cutting This is sometimes called 'scissor tapering'. This technique is often used in barbering to blend heavier sections of hair into shorter hair, such as may be found on some men with male pattern baldness. It is usually achieved by moving the scissor blades along the hair in a slithering or sliding movement when it reduces weight at the ends of the section without affecting the overall length.

SMARTER objectives A management acronym used to describe how objectives should be written:
Specific;
Measureable;
Achieveable;
Realistic;
Timebound;
Evaluated;
Resourced.

Stylist This term can also include technicians, specialists and product demonstrators.

Tapered necklines Tapered necklines have soft outlines that follow the natural hairline shape so that the nape outline appears to fade out with no harsh lines visible.

Thinning Reducing the amount of hair without reducing the length. Within the standards at Level 2, this will be carried out with scissors. The use of razors for thinning is included in appropriate Level 3 standards.

Tonging A technique that uses any heated equipment that traps hair to change its structure (e.g. Marcell type tongs, crimpers and spring tongs).

Tools Refers to any tools necessary to deliver a hairdressing service.

Traditional looks A man's look that has been established and popular over a long period of time e.g. a crew cut.

Tree plaiting Plaiting that leaves stems of hair protruding down the length of the plait at regular and even intervals.

Unconventional items Refers to items such as foil, straws, chopsticks, rik rak, etc, that can be used for setting hair to create different, creative effects in hair.

Virgin hair Hair that has not had any chemical treatment on it.

White hair (i.e. Canities) The term used to describe colourless hair, commonly known as grey hair.

Workplace This word is used to describe the single or multiple areas in which you carry out your work. Normally, this will be your salon.

Workplace policies This covers the documentation prepared by your employer on the procedures to be followed in your workplace. Examples are your employer's safety policy statement, or general health and safety statements and written safety procedures covering aspects of the workplace that should be drawn to the employees' (and 'other persons') attention, pricing policies and customer service policies.

Working practices Any activities, procedures, use of materials or equipment and working techniques used in carrying out your job. Lifting techniques and maintaining good posture whilst working are also included.

Yarn locks Locks created by wrapping wool, thread and/or string around the length of the hair.

GENERAL GUIDANCE ON HEALTH AND SAFETY LEGISLATION APPLICABLE TO HAIRDRESSING

Health and Safety is the responsibility of all persons at work. Employers and supervisors in particular have a greater responsibility for health and safety than, say, the trainee stylist or stylist, but **all** have a responsibility to work in a healthy and safe manner.

Section 7 of the Health and Safety at Work Act of 1974 states:

'It shall be the duty of every employee while at work:

1 to take reasonable care for the health and safety of himself and of other persons who may be affected by his acts or omissions at work;

and

2 as regard any duty or requirement imposed on the employer or any other person by or under any of the relevant statutory provisions, to co-operate with him so far as is necessary to enable that duty or requirement to be performed or complied with'.

There are many individual items of health and safety legislation that apply to the working of a hairdressing salon. Some, like 'The Management of Health and Safety at Work Regulations 1992' (which require management to carry out a Risk Assessment of their salons, to identify hazards and to improve working conditions and practices) obviously apply mainly to your employer. Other items of legislation apply to employers **and** all those working within the salon.

The following are the principle items of legislation that apply to general salon operations and, therefore, to employers **and** employees/trainees, etc, alike:

1 The Health and Safety at Work etc. Act 1974 is the great 'enabling' Act from which most of the subsequent legislation has sprung.

2 The Workplace (Health Safety & Welfare) Regulations 1992 have taken the place of most of the Office, Shops and Railway Premises Act 1963, and require all at work to help maintain a safe and healthy working environment. They apply very much to hairdressing salons.

3 The Manual Handling Operations Regulations 1992 places upon all at work the duty to minimise the risks from lifting and handling objects.

4 The Provision and Use of Work Equipment Regulations 1992 impose upon the employee the duty to select equipment for use at work which is properly constructed, suitable for the purpose and kept in good repair. Employers must also ensure that all who use the equipment have been adequately trained. The requirement for competence to use salon tools and equipment is embodied within the hairdressing standards.

5 The Personal Protective Equipment at Work Regulations 1992 confirm the requirement for employers to provide suitable and sufficient protective clothing/equipment, and for all employees to use it when required. The use of Personal Protective Equipment (PPE) is a requirement of the hairdressing standards.

6 The Control of Substances Hazardous to Health Regulations 1992 (often referred to as COSHH) to include subsequent amendments are particularly important as the storage, use and sale of a wide range of chemicals forms an important part of salon services, especially as such substances are applied on and sold to non-employees, i.e. clients.

7 The Electricity at Work Regulations 1989. Under this law, your salon is required to maintain electrical equipment in a safe condition. It is your responsibility to report any faulty electrical equipment that you come across in your workplace.

8 Reporting of Injuries, Diseases and Dangerous Occurrences Regulations 1985 (often referred to as RIDDOR). Under this regulation, your salon is required to report injuries, disease and dangerous occurrences. It is your responsibility to report to the relevant person any injuries and dangerous occurrences that happen at work. Your salon may also require you to report potentially infectious conditions of which you become aware.

9 Cosmetic Products (Safety) Regulations 1989. This law lays down rules for recommended volumes and strengths of different hydroxide-based products. The strength of a product will vary depending on whether it has been prepared for professional or non-professional general use. It is important that when using these products, you check its strength from the manufacturer's guidance notes and check current legislation. (Copies of the Regulations can be bought from Her Majesty's Stationery Office (HMSO) bookshops. Guidance can also be obtained from individual manufacturers and the Hairdressing and Beauty Suppliers Association.)

RANGE OF SERVICE TIMES FOR LEVEL 3 HAIRDRESSING SERVICES

Owing to the nature of many of the services in the proposed Level 3 NVQ/SVQ, it is not possible to set a precise time for completion. Times for critical aspects of various services are quoted below.

Service	Style	Maximum time (minutes)
1. Perm winding only	a. piggy back	Maximum
	b. spiral	45
	c. weaving	90
	d. stack	45
	e. root	45
	f. hopscotch	25
	g. double	45
2. Colour application (all methods in range)		45
3. Thermal pressing (straightening)		45
4. Thermal styling (excluding spiral curls)		30
5. Relaxer application and removal		30
6. Face massage		20

INDEX